NUTRITION
for a
HEALTHY MOUTH

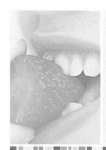

NUTRITION
for a
HEALTHY MOUTH

Rebecca Sroda, RDH, MS
Director of Dental Education
South Florida Community College
Avon Park, Florida

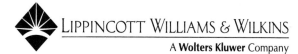

LIPPINCOTT WILLIAMS & WILKINS
A **Wolters Kluwer** Company

Philadelphia · Baltimore · New York · London
Buenos Aires · Hong Kong · Sydney · Tokyo

Acquisitions Editor: John Goucher
Managing Editor: Kevin C. Dietz
Marketing Manager: Hilary Henderson
Production Editor: Sirkka E.H. Bertling
Designer: Risa Clow
Compositor: Maryland Composition, Inc.
Printer: R.R. Donnelly & Sons (Crawfordsville)

Printed in the United States of America

Library of Congress Cataloging-in-Publication Data

Sroda, Rebecca.
    Nutrition for a healthy mouth / Rebecca Sroda.
        p. ; cm.
    Includes bibliographical references and index.
    ISBN 0-7817-5155-1
1. Nutrition and dental health.   2. Mouth—Diseases—Nutritional aspects.   3. Dental assistants.
4. Nutrition. I. Title.
    [DNLM: 1. Mouth Diseases—diet therapy. 2. Dental Assistants. 3. Nutrition. 4. Oral Hygiene.   ]
RK281.S67 2005
617.6'01—dc22

                                              2004022704

05 06 07 08 09
1 2 3 4 5 6 7 8 9 10

*This book is dedicated to Jill Nield-Gehrig,
mentor-extraordinaire!*

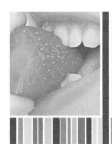

PREFACE

How to Use This Book

This book is intended to serve as both textbook and reference for three groups of users: dental assisting students, dental hygiene students, and practicing clinicians.

Readers of this book will find it designed in such a way that the study of nutrition can be individualized depending on the depth of instruction required for the different classes of students or the specific need of the patient.

- For dental hygiene students who take but one nutrition class, this book can serve as an all-encompassing text for both a general and dental-related study of nutrition.

- Dental hygiene students who take a general nutrition class before enrolling in the dental-related course will find this book useful for a quick review of basic nutrition before embarking on an in-depth study of dental nutritional counseling.

- Dental assisting students, whose curriculum allows for only a few weeks of nutritional study, may glean topics from chapters to cover information required in their curriculum.

Further reading sections and recommended websites are included at the end of each chapter for those who wish to conduct a more in-depth study of a particular topic.

Information is organized into seven major sections:

Section I: Introduction

Section II: Major Nutrients

Section III: Relationship of Nutrition to Oral Disease

Section IV: Food Guidelines

Section V: Food for Growth

Section VI: Nutritional Counseling
Appendices

The laminated redi-reference card is intended to be used at chairside during patient education to help patients associate daily nutrition with dental caries and periodontal disease. Seventy-five percent of what we learn is through the sense of sight, and these guides will enhance information sessions to have more of a lasting impact.

Each chapter has activities that allow the reader to "work" with the information and give the subject a practical application. Students should be encouraged to fill in the blanks and complete work sheets. Chapter quizzes can be used as weekly quizzes or as preparation for more in-depth examinations.

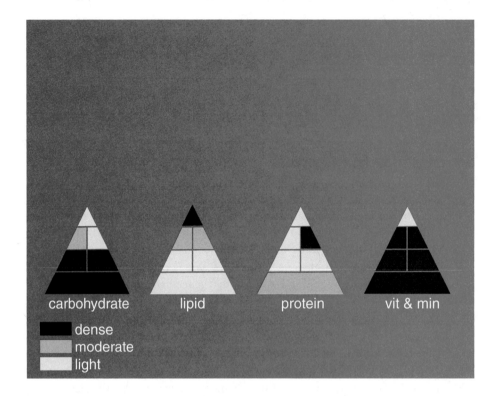

A "Putting This Into Practice" section functions as a vehicle for students to critically think about topics covered and to give significance to daily food choices for both the text user and patient.

Counseling suggestions are offered at the end of each major nutrient chapter to remedy deficiencies in a particular food group. After having a patient complete a food diary and analyzing strengths and weaknesses, the reader can turn to the end of the major nutrient chapter for ideas to help patients improve their food selection. Look for the food pyramid with gradient degrees of shading to indicate which food groups contain the specific nutrient.

The forms section (Appendix III) as well as suggestions for counseling patients with deficiencies makes dental nutritional counseling quick and easy to incorporate into patient treatment.

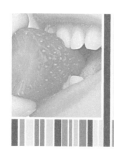

TABLE OF CONTENTS

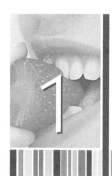

EATING 101

It is not what you choose to eliminate from your diet that makes it healthy, but rather what you choose to include.

Introduction

Meal planning, preparation, and eating are very different in the 21st century than they were in the last, which has made our lives unique from previous generations. We have mutated the concept of family mealtime with the help of food processing plants, the fast food industry, and mass marketing concepts.[1,2] The emergence of frozen dinners has increased the popularity of a massive food processing industry, which gives us a new way to "restaurant" and allows "cooks" to broaden their horizons. Mom is no longer in the kitchen baking cookies when the kids come home from school, and dinner is not always on the table when the "bread winner" returns home after a long, hard day at work. Families now find themselves without a chief cook in the kitchen and consuming 65% of all meals in their cars. When we order a meal from a restaurant, four out of five times we are sitting in a car.[3] We stop and pick up breakfast on our way to work, grab a quick bite for lunch, and stop for fast food in the evening before getting to our final destination. We can drink breakfast from a bottle, eat lunch out of a box, and eat dinner from a carton. Gone are the days when the whole family gathers around a beautifully set table, at the same time everyday, partaking of a meal that took two hours to prepare. Fine civilized dining is reserved only for special occasions.

When we view the Food Pyramid, we have to look at it through the eyes of someone living in the 21st century: we have to remember that all those pictures of delicious looking fruits and vegetables are not out back ready to be picked off the vine or tree, that bread is not baking in the oven, and that we don't eat "three square meals" a day. We are very busy people; this is where our patients are coming from, and where we must meet them.

We need to consider the trends in the 21st century as we guide our patients to choose food wisely. The following list includes some of these trends: [2,4,5]

- We have a tendency to eat on the run.
- People are surpassing the life expectancy age, creating a vast aging population with their own unique set of health problems.
- Adult obesity has doubled in the last 20 years.
- Even though we are more aware of the benefits of daily exercise we remain sedentary, spending more time in front of the TV or computer.
- More hours per day are spent at work, putting more stress on the body.

Food Choices and Nutrient Needs

Nutrition is what we choose to eat and put into our bodies, and the food we select contains nutrients—chemical substances that provide the body with energy and everything else it needs to function. Ninety-six percent of human body mass is comprised of the elements oxygen, carbon, hydrogen, and nitrogen. These elements also make up the six major nutrients found in food, making the saying "you are what you eat" really ring true.[6] We need to eat every day to provide the body with a steady supply of fuel, which is created by digestion and absorption of six major nutrients: carbohydrates, proteins, lipids, water, vitamins, and minerals. Often, our bodies, in their own subtle way, will let us know which foods to choose to get the necessary nutrients. When we are dehydrated, we thirst for water (hydrogen and oxygen); when our activity level increases, we crave protein (carbon, hydrogen, oxygen, and nitrogen); and when we increase our mental activity, we crave carbohydrates (carbon, hydrogen, and oxygen). The six major nutrients are detailed in Box 1-1.

The first thing that usually comes to mind when thinking of a nutrient is one or two specific foods from the predominant food group. For example, we think of something sweet for carbohydrates, or meat and eggs for protein. The fact is, most foods contain all six of the major nutrients. The proportion of the nutrients to each other in a specific food is what gives the food a label of either "carbohydrate rich," "protein rich," or "high fat."

The food choices we make each day should be well thought out to keep our bodies healthy and performing efficiently. Eating too much of any one thing will usually

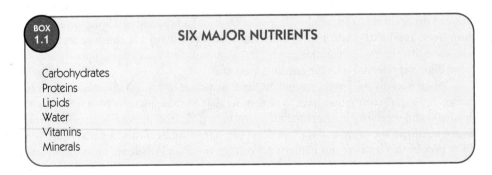

BOX 1.1

SIX MAJOR NUTRIENTS

Carbohydrates
Proteins
Lipids
Water
Vitamins
Minerals

"squeeze out" other food choices. For example, daily consumption of fast foods decreases the chance of consuming more wholesomely prepared foods, and eating sweets throughout the day leaves less appetite for healthier snacks. This is not to say that we should never eat these foods; we just should not eat them exclusively every day or for weeks on end.

The relationship between food and the disease process happens when the body gets too much or too little of a particular nutrient over a period of time. Diabetes, heart disease, and colon, breast, and reproductive cancers are a few of the major diseases associated with unhealthy eating habits.[7–11] Consistently making unhealthy food choices can cause a major disease and a shorter lifespan. The lesson here is that, as humans, we can eat almost anything and still remain healthy, as long as it is in moderation.

The Food Pyramid

The U.S. Department of Agriculture (USDA) Food Pyramid, shown in Figure 1-1, was designed as a guide to healthy eating and to making healthy food choices.

Serving suggestions for six food groups have been made to ensure a daily supply of important nutrients. It should be remembered that the Food Pyramid guidelines are suggestions and can be modified to accommodate specific diet requirements, such as those for people who are vegetarians, who are lactose intolerant, or who have specific cultural

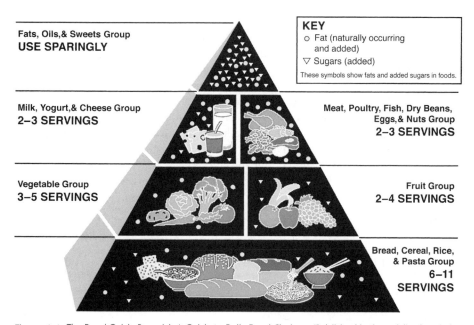

Figure 1-1. The Food Guide Pyramid: A Guide to Daily Food Choices. (Published in the public domain by the U.S. Department of Agriculture and the U.S. Department of Health and Human Services. 5th ed. 2000.)

and religious practices. According to the Food Pyramid, we should include a variety of foods from each category, considering the following while doing so:

- Three rich sources of calcium
- Three high protein foods
- At least five servings of vegetables and fruits
- Whole grains for fiber
- Vegetable fats and omega-3 fat

Add to that at least eight glasses of water and moderate exercise, and you have a plan to maintain a healthy body. (See Chapter 11 for more detail on the Food Pyramid.)

Food Habits

We may be choosing the food we eat out of habit or because we have a physiologic need for certain nutrients. Some food habits have multiple origins. They can be born out of family traditions—like turkey for Thanksgiving, cake on birthdays, and cookies for Christmas. Other habits are created because of the way food makes us feel, especially when we are stressed or upset. Foods high in fat and carbohydrates tend to be chosen as comfort foods.[12-14] A physiologic need for certain foods—also considered a craving—can turn into a true habit if not met. Social occasions add to our habits with their cyclic list of foods to serve, for example, veggies and dip, sushi, and other finger foods. Box 1-2 lists some sources of food habits.

Reasons for Food Habits

It has been said that our bodies have an innate wisdom and will let us know when they need something, and that when we have a craving our bodies are talking to us. Whether or not this is true, the fact is that food cravings can be either physiologic or emotional. Not everybody gets them, but for those who do, they are very real. Hormone fluctuation can trigger a food craving, which is why they are reported more by women than men.[15, 16] Cravings can turn into a full-blown habit that needs to be fed on a daily basis. Sometimes they are a steady constant, like having ice cream every night after dinner. We can go through phases, like eating peanut butter and crackers every day around 4:00 PM for two weeks, and then smoked almonds at the same time for the next two weeks. This is nei-

BOX 1.2

REASONS FOR FOOD HABITS

Cultural
Traditional
Emotional
Physiological
Social

ther accidental nor coincidental. If what we crave is based on a physiologic need, then our bodies will let us know when they are balanced and no longer need the chemical. If our craving is on an emotional level, then the craving remains as long as the emotional need remains. If we fulfill the need, then the craving goes away.

What are our bodies trying to tell us when we have a craving? Usually one of four things:

1. We need a mood adjustment—levels of neurotransmitters are fluctuating and we need to balance them with a nutrient in the specific food we crave.
2. Our blood sugar is low and we need carbohydrates to boost our energy level.
3. We are lacking a specific nutrient and the food we crave will balance our chemistry.
4. Something is out of balance emotionally and we need a comfort food to help us cope.

Here are some ideas to minimize a food craving:

- Move your body—exercise, stretch, or practice yoga to stave off depressive feelings.
- Choose complex carbohydrates for meals that will moderate blood sugar levels throughout the day.
- Eat frequent small nutritious meals throughout the day. This will keep you from becoming overly hungry.
- Give in and eat a modest amount of what you crave.

Chocolate is the single-most craved food.[17] Some say it isn't even food, but rather medicine. It contains phenylethylamine, a mood enhancer, and caffeinelike substances called methylxanthine and theobromine. Eating chocolate balances brain chemicals and boosts energy.

Take a moment and think about your reasons for eating the foods you do. Pay attention to your body to determine if specific foods can change how you feel. When you feel like eating a snack, such as potato chips or candy, ask yourself if you are truly hungry, or if you are bored, upset, anxious, or tired. Identifying the feeling before you eat can help you understand your eating habits. Complete Table 1-1 and see if foods you choose affect you in a certain way.

Review of the Digestive System

The gastrointestinal (GI) tract, which supplies the body with nutrients and water, includes the following organs:

1. esophagus
2. stomach
3. small intestine
4. large intestine
5. rectum

Table 1-1. Influence of Food

Keep a record of how your food selections make you feel. Check in with your body 30 minutes after consuming a particular food to determine what it does.

Food	Energetic	Happy	Clear mind	Disoriented	Sleepy	Depressed
1						
2						
3						
4						
5						
6						
7						
8						
9						
10						

Three other organs—the pancreas, liver, and gallbladder—secrete enzymes that help reduce the food to micronutrients. Carbohydrates are reduced to monosaccharides, a source of fuel for the body, with the help of salivary and pancreatic *amylase*. The pancreas also secretes *lipase* and the liver and gallbladder produce *bile*; all of these aid with the digestion of fats. The entire digestive system is illustrated in Figure 1-2.

Food's journey begins in the mouth, where chewing reduces it to smaller particles, making it easier to swallow and pass through to the stomach. The human dentition crushes food with a force of almost 200 pounds (90 kg), mashing and mixing the bolus of food with saliva and the enzyme amylase and splitting starch molecules into smaller units. Swallowing pushes the food into the **esophagus**, the "hallway" that funnels food into the stomach by way of peristalsis (alternating contractions and relaxation), until it hits the sphincter, the "door" that will open and admit the food to the stomach.

The **stomach** stores the masticated food for about an hour and a half and continues to break it down into smaller particles with the stomach enzyme *pepsinogen* and *hydrochloric acid*, which is secreted by the gastric gland. At this point, the liver produces *bile* to break down fat molecules, and protein begins to be digested. The contents being

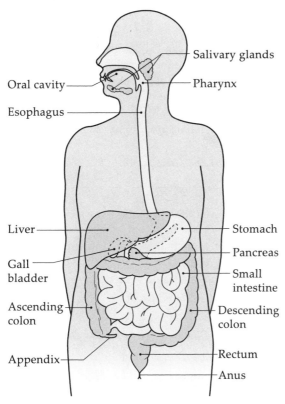

Figure 1-2. The digestive system.

held in the stomach—food bolus, enzymes, bile, and acids—have been turned into a mixture called chyme, which continues the journey into the intestines. Proteins, starches, fats, vitamins, minerals, water, and alcohol have all been reduced to the smallest unit possible so they can permeate the intestinal wall and find their way into the bloodstream.

The **small intestine** is divided into three sections: duodenum, jejunum, and ileum. Most digestion takes place in the small intestines, more specifically the jejunum. The lining of the intestines is variegated rather than smooth, with peaks called villi. The villi extensions increase the surface area of the small intestines, allowing for quicker passage of nutrients (3 to 10 hours). Once these small units of digested food pass into the bloodstream, they travel to all parts of the body, supplying it with fuel and nutrients needed for all metabolic processes.

Remnants of food that didn't digest become waste and pass on to the **large intestine**, where water is absorbed from the waste, turning it to solid feces. Unlike the small intestine, the lining of the large intestine is smooth. Bacteria in the feces can manufacture vitamin D and Biotin, which can be absorbed and used by the body.

The **rectum** stores the feces until our brain gets the signal to eliminate it. Total "intestinal transit time" can be anywhere from 24 hours to 3 weeks.

What Is in the Future?

Have you noticed that two people can eat exactly the same food, in exactly the same amount, and one person maintains an ideal weight and the other becomes obese? The reason for this is that we are all chemically different. Scientists say our genes determine which nutrients get absorbed and metabolized and which don't. With a small drop of blood, nutritional genomics labs can analyze your DNA and develop a designer diet that will balance individual micro- and macronutrient needs and keep your body healthy.

PUTTING THIS INTO PRACTICE

The goal of this project is to jump-start your mind to begin thinking about nutrition and its relationship to the body.

Your assignment is to visit a grocery store of your choice with a relative or friend and passively observe their food choices and food selection process.

Answer the following questions about your observations:

1. List the food items in your selected person's shopping cart.

2. What body type do they have? Circle one:

   Ectomorphic—light body build with slight muscular development

   Mesomorphic—husky muscular body build

   Endomorphic—heavy rounded body build often with a marked tendency to become fat

3. Does their body type match the food they have chosen to eat? Explain.

4. Who or what do you think they were shopping for?

5. What would you add to their selection to balance out their diet?

6. What would you eliminate from their selection to make their diet more nutritious?

7. Did they read labels as they chose food for their carts?

8. Draw a conclusion about food choices and our bodies.

Web Resources

American Dietetic Association (ADA)
www.eatright.org

The Blonz Guide to Nutrition, Food Science, and Health www.blonz.com

CDC's Nutrition and Physical Activity
www.cdc.gov/nccdphp/dnpa

ENC: Egg Nutrition Center
www.enc-online.org

Food and Nutrition Information Center
www.nal.usda.gov/fnic

Government Information on Nutrition
www.nutrition.gov

Harvard School of Public Health
www.hsph.harvard.edu

Journal of Nutrition www.nutrition.org

Nutrition Action Health Letter
www.cspinet.org/nah/index.htm

Nutrition and Healthy Eating Advice
www.nutrition.about.com

Tufts University Nutrition Navigator: A Rating Guide to Nutrition Websites
www.navigator.tufts.edu

Untangling the Web—How to Find Useful Nutrition and Health Information On Line http://cspinet.org/nah/2003/untangling_the_web.html

The Vegetarian Resource Group
www.vrg.org/nutrition

References

1. Schlosser E. Fast Food Nation: The Dark Side of the All American Meal. Boston: Houghton Mifflin, 2000.

2. Popkin BM. Nutrition in transition: the changing global nutrition challenge. Asia Pac J Clin Nutr. 2001;10(Suppl):S13–18.

3. Blake J. Measuring our dining, shopping habits—survey finds we like to eat out, shop around (survey from Market Research Firm NPD Foodworld). Seattle Times, Feb. 11, 2003.

4. Ebbin R. American's dining out habits. Restaurants USA, November 2000.

5. Tougher-Decker R, Mobley CC, American Dietetic Association. Position of the American Dietetic Association: oral health and nutrition. J Am Diet Assoc. 2003;103(5):615–625.

6. Katch FI, Katch VL, McArdle WD. Introduction to Nutrition, Exercise, and Health. 4th Ed. Baltimore: Lippincott Williams and Wilkins, 1993.

7. Key TJ, Schatzkin A, Willett WC, Allen NE, Spencer EA, Travis RC. Diet, nutrition and the prevention of cancer. Public Health Nutr. 2004;7(1A):187–200.

8. Vandewater EA, Shim MS, Caplovitz AG. Linking obesity and activity level with children's television and video game use. J Adolesc. 2004;27(1): 71–85.

9. Simonpoulos AP. The traditional diet of Greece and cancer. Eur J Cancer Prev. 2004;13:219–230.

10. Cannon G. Why the Bush administration and the global sugar industry are determined to demolish the 2004 WHO global strategy on diet, physical activity and health. Public Health Nutr. 2004;7(3):369–380.

11. Proietto J, Baur LA. 10: Management of obesity. Med J Aust. 2004;180 (9):474–480.

12. Pelchat ML. Of human bondage: food craving, obsession, compulsion, and addiction. Physiol Behav. 2002;76(3):347–352.

13. Yanovski S. Sugar and fat: cravings and aversions. J Nutr. 2003;133(3): 835S–837S.

14. Cramwinckel B. Feeling like a snack. The influence of taste on our eating habits. Ned Tijdschr Tandheelkd. 1995;102(11):435–437.

15. Michener W, Rozin P, Freeman E, et al. The role of low progesterone and tension as triggers of perimenstrual chocolate and sweets craving: some negative experimental evidence. Physiol Behav. 1999;67(3):417–420.

16. Kurzer MS. Women, food and mood. Nutr Rev. 1997;55(7):268–276.

17. Bruinsma K, Taren DL. Chocolate: food or drug? J Am Diet Assoc. 1999;99(10):1249–1256.

Suggested Readings

Christensen L, Pettijohn L. Mood and carbohydrate cravings. Appetite 2001;36 (2):137–145.

Ehrlich A. Nutrition and Dental Health, 2nd Ed. Albany: Delmar Learning, 1994.

Hill AJ, Weaver CF, Blundell JE. Food craving, dietary restraint and mood. Appetite 1991;17(3):187–197.

Matthiessen J, Fagt S, Biltoft-Jensen A, Beck AM, Ovesen L. Size makes a difference. Public Health Nutr. 2003;6(1): 65–72.

Smiciklas-Wright H, Mitchell DC, Mickle SJ, Goldman JD, Cook A. Foods commonly eaten in the United States, 1989-1991 and 1994-1996: are portion sizes changing? J Am Diet Assoc. 2003;103 (1):39–40.

Wansink B, Cheney MM, Chan N. Exploring comfort food preferences across age and gender. Physiol Behav. 2003;79(4–5):739–747.

Weingarten HP, Elston D. The phenomenology of food cravings. Appetite 1990;15(3):231–246.

Wilson N, Quigley R, Mansoor O. Food ads on TV: a health hazard for children? Aust NZ J Public Health. 1999;23 (6):647–650.

Zellner DA, Garriga-Trillo A, Rohm E, Centeno S, Parker S. Food liking and craving: a cross-cultural approach. Appetite 1999;33(1):61–70.

SECTION II: Major Nutrients

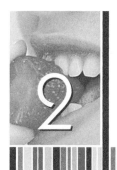

CARBOHYDRATES

The Body's Fuel

Before the Industrial Revolution, carbohydrates (CHO) were the greatest proportion of foods consumed and therefore the main source of nutrients. Geographically, regions had their own **staple food** that was indigenous to their land. These carbohydrates were consumed in their whole or natural form (without processing) and considered rich with vitamins, minerals, and fiber. Table 2-1 identifies the food staple by region.

Along with the Industrial Revolution came the invention of a machine for everything, including for processing wheat, sugarcane, and sugar beets into a refined white powder. To get the fine white powder, the husks and pulp had to be removed, which was the part of the plant that contained all the nutrients and fiber. Because these were removed, the powdered flour and sugar lost nutritive value but retained calories. It was considered a luxury and a display of wealth to have a pantry full of bleached white flour and sugar, and its owner usually had a growing belly to prove it. What once were wealthy sources of nutrients became poor sources, but the consumption of them remained the

Table 2-1. Main Food Staples by Region	
Asia	Rice
Middle East	Wheat
Great Britain	Barley and oats
Pacific Islands	Taro root
Africa	Cassava root and yams
America	Potatoes and corn

same. People began to load their meals with "refined" ingredients, which corresponded to an increase in incidence of obesity. Accusations were made that all carbohydrates were fattening. This has since been proved false because it was discovered that all the "extras" eaten with the meal, not the carbohydrates, caused the increase in obesity. Butter, sour cream, salad dressing, and added sugars such as jellies, jams, and syrup are now recognized as the fat-producing culprits. Carbohydrates, when carefully selected, can actually be an excellent low-fat source of fiber and nutrients.

When asked, most people will reply that carbohydrates are sugar. In essence, they are half right. Carbohydrates are a *type* of sugar, but all carbohydrates are not sweet like table sugar. Rice, pasta, bread, fruits, and vegetables are also considered carbohydrates. The size of the molecule is what determines the flavor, but they all do pretty much the same thing in the body.

Primary Role of Carbohydrates in the Body

The primary roles of carbohydrates are to:

- Supply the body with energy
- Maintain blood glucose levels
- Continue brain and nervous system function, even while sleeping
- Spare protein so the body does not burn dietary or body fat and protein for energy
- Burn fat for fuel
- Provide bulk in the diet (fiber) and keep you full

Source of Carbohydrates

The word "carbohydrate" is Latin for hydrated water. Carbohydrates are often abbreviated to CHO for the three elements that compose it: carbon, hydrogen, and oxygen. The chemical building blocks of CHOs are called monosaccharides, which are composed of six carbon atoms and six water molecules.

With the exception of one sugar, plants are the source of all carbohydrates. Figure 2-1 illustrates where CHOs fit into the food chain.

Food Chain

1. Plant roots absorb water.
2. Foliage absorbs carbon dioxide (CO_2) from the air.
3. Plant absorbs rays from the sun.
4. Chloroplasts in the plant take all three—H_2O, sun, and CO_2—and through photosynthesis make monosaccharides.
5. Animals eat the plant and reduce the monosaccharides to glucose.

Box 2-1 identifies the only CHO of animal origin.

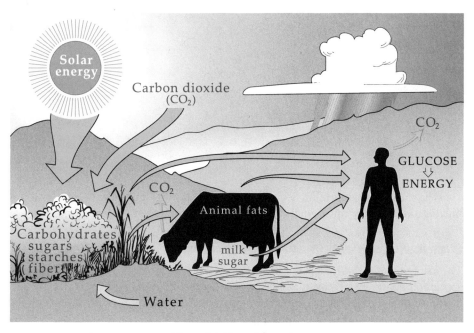

Figure 2-1. The carbon cycle.

| BOX 2.1 | LACTOSE |

Lactose (milk sugar) is the only carbohydrate of animal origin.

Classification of Carbohydrates

Generally speaking, there are two ways to classify CHOs: Table 2-2 outlines these two classification systems.

Table 2-2. Classification of Carbohydrates

Chemical	Nutritional
Monosaccharide	Simple carbohydrate
Disaccharide	
Oligosaccharide	Complex carbohydrate
Polysaccharide	

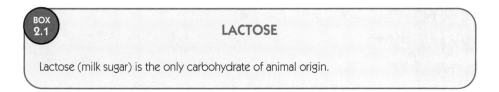

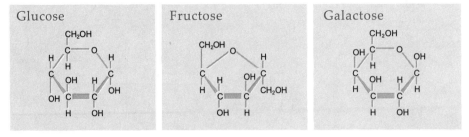

Figure 2-2. Chemical structure of monosaccharides.

The chemical classification helps us understand how the molecules of carbohydrates link together, and the nutritional classification determines their value in our diet.

Chemical Classification of Carbohydrates

The main unit of carbohydrate is a glucose molecule. One molecule of glucose consists of six carbon atoms, 12 hydrogen atoms, and six oxygen atoms: $C_6H_{12}O_6$. Figures 2-2 and 2-3 illustrate the chemical structures of monosaccharides and disaccharides, respectively.

1. Monosaccharide: one molecule of sugar
2. Disaccharide: two molecules of sugar
3. Oligosaccharide: two to 10 molecules of sugar
4. Polysaccharide: more than 10 molecules of sugar

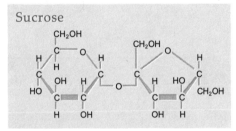

Nutritional Classification of Carbohydrates

Simple Sugars

Monosaccharides and disaccharides are referred to as simple sugars. Foods that are considered simple sugars are usually those that are sweet to the taste. Candy, cookies, cake, soda, ripe fruits, and other baked goods fall in this category and are high in calories but lack the nutrients supplied by complex carbohydrates. Milk and glucose (blood sugar) are also considered simple sugars, but are not sweet to the taste.

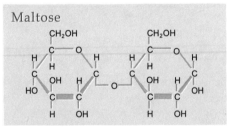

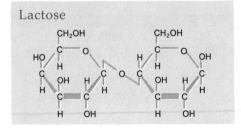

Figure 2-3. Chemical structure of disaccharides.

BOX 2.2

MONOSACCHARIDES

- Glucose—blood sugar
- Fructose—fruit sugar
- Galactose—milk

Box 2-2 lists common monosaccharides and Box 2-3 lists common disaccharides.

Monosaccharides:

1. Glucose (also called dextrose or blood sugar) is the main currency for the body's fuel source that supplies energy. Most other sugars are either converted or broken down to this unit. Glucose can be stored as glycogen in muscle and the liver, or if consumed in excess, can be converted to fat for future energy supply.
2. Fructose is the sweetest of all sugars and found in fruit and honey. It is converted by the body to glucose.
3. Galactose, also known as milk sugar, is converted by the body to glucose.

Disaccharides:

1. Sucrose (also known as table sugar) consists of the monosaccharides glucose and fructose, which make table sugar sweet. This is used in cooking and baking for a sweet taste.
2. Maltose consists of two glucose molecules and is created when larger carbohydrate molecules are broken down during digestion.
3. Lactose, the sugar found in milk, splits into the two monosaccharides glucose and galactose during digestion.

Complex Carbohydrates

Polysaccharides are referred to as complex carbohydrates. Foods high in complex carbohydrates contain vitamins, minerals, fiber, and water. Brown rice, whole grain bread, cereal, whole wheat pasta, legumes, fruits, and vegetables are foods rich in complex car-

BOX 2.3

DISACCHARIDES

- Sucrose—glucose + fructose = table sugar
- Maltose—glucose + glucose = flavoring, breakdown product of starch
- Lactose—glucose + galactose = milk disaccharide

BOX 2.4

POLYSACCHARIDES

- Oligosaccharide
- Starch
- Glycogen
- Fiber

bohydrates. Complex carbohydrates supply more nutrients than simple carbohydrates and are a very good low-fat food source. Box 2-4 lists common polysaccharides.

The following list corresponds with polysaccharides listed in Box 2-4:

1. Oligosaccharides

   Oligosaccharides are a unique type of carbohydrate because the body does not metabolize them in the usual way. They are larger than a disaccharide—at least two or more single sugar molecules—and are found in legumes (beans). Oligosaccharides pass through the stomach undigested into the intestines, where bacteria feed on the carbohydrate and create a gaseous end-product (which gives beans their bad reputation).

2. Starch

   Starch is the storage form of energy in plants, just as glycogen is the storage form of energy in animals. The arrangement of glucose molecules determines whether the starch is amylose or amylopectin, the two most predominant starches.

BOX 2.5

FILL IN THE BLANKS:

_____is to animals as _____is to plants.

Amylopectin is a series of highly branched chains of glucose molecules. It is sometimes referred to as a waxy starch that forms a stringy paste when heated, and this property makes it work well as a thickener in food. Amylose is comprised of thousands of straight-chain glucose molecules. Foods that contain starch are grains, legumes, tubers (potatoes, yams, turnips), and some fruits.

BOX 2.6

A fancy name for starch is dextrose.

> ## Table 2-3. Simple Carbohydrates and Complex Carbohydrates
>
> | Simple Carbohydrate | Complex Carbohydrate |
> | --- | --- |
> | White bread | Whole grain bread |
> | White rice | Brown rice |
> | Semolina pasta | Whole wheat pasta |
> | Sugar-sweetened juices | 100% fruit and vegetable juice |
> | Flour tortillas | Wheat or spinach tortillas |

See which foods you eat contain starch by performing the simple experiment detailed in Box 2-7.

Function of Starches

Starch is used as a thickening agent in cooking and baking. A good example is corn-starch: When mixed with water over heat, it forms a sauce or gravy. When we consume starch, it gives us a sense of *satiety* or fullness, and the sense of being full stays with us for a longer period of time.

Digestion of Starch

- Salivary amylase in the mouth breaks starch down to dextrins.
- Pancreatic amylase in the small intestine breaks dextrins down to maltose.
- Maltase splits maltose into glucose units, which can be absorbed.
3. Glycogen

   Glycogen is the most highly branched chain of glucose units and is the storage form of carbohydrates that is found in the liver and muscle.

   In liver—helps maintain blood glucose levels

   In muscle—provides quick supply of energy for muscles

BOX 2.7

EXPERIMENT WITH YOUR FOOD

One way to tell if a food contains starch is to add a drop of iodine. The unbranched helical shape of amylose reacts strongly to iodine and turns it blue-black. Amylopectin, cellulose, and glycogen will turn the iodine reddish-purple and brown.

4. Fiber

Fiber is the food that is usually referred to as *roughage* or *bulk* and is not used by the body for energy. Fiber is thousands of glucose units bonded together and is found exclusively in plants, giving them structure. Fiber in plants is equal to bones in animals. A good example of fiber is the stringy strips that run the length of celery.

Humans do not have enzymes that can break down and digest fiber. The chemical links between fiber molecules are joined in such a way that they cannot be separated by human digestive enzymes. Vitamins and minerals in fiber-rich foods are not made available to the body and pass through unabsorbed.

Two Classes of Fiber

Soluble Fiber—dissolves in water

- Examples are gums, mucilage, and pectin, as in the gelatinous substance that forms in cooked oatmeal.
- Foods high in soluble fiber are fruits, vegetables, grains, beans, oats, and apples

Function of Soluble Fiber

- Adds chewy or crunchy texture to foods
- Gives a sense of satiety—keeps the stomach full longer
- Stabilizes blood sugar—takes longer for the body to metabolize and slows release of glucose into bloodstream
- Helps lower cholesterol—binds fiber and carries it out of the body in waste

Insoluble Fiber—does not dissolve in water

- Insoluble fiber is found in seeds.
- Other examples are cellulose and lignin, like the stringy strips in celery. Cellulose is the most abundant polysaccharide.
- Foods high in insoluble fiber are vegetables, whole grains, wheat bran, and apples.

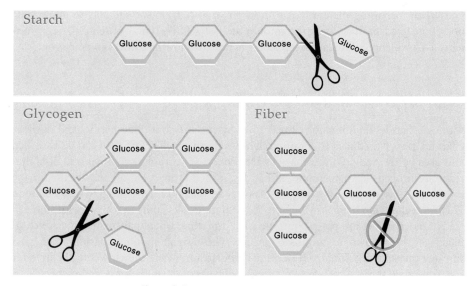

Figure 2-4. Enzymes cannot break apart fiber.

Function of Insoluble Fiber

Insoluble fiber prevents disease by stimulating peristalsis and keeps colon muscles exercised and strong. Fiber also acts to decrease:

- constipation
- hemorrhoids
- diverticulosis (outpouchings in colon wall)/diverticulitis (infected outpouchings)
- colon cancer—empties the colon so that lining of intestines and colon are not exposed to toxins for a long period of time
- incidence of appendicitis

Table 2-4. Grams of Fiber in Food

Food	Total Fiber	Soluble Fiber	Insoluble Fiber
Oat bran	28	14	14
Rolled oats	14	8	6
Wheat bran	43	3	40
Kidney beans	10	5	5
Pinto beans	11	5	6
Corn	3	2	1
Apple	2	1	1
Orange	2	1	1

When increasing the amount of fiber in your diet, do so gradually to allow your body time to adapt. Increasing the amount too fast will result in waste elimination problems. Drink plenty of fluids to keep stools hydrated, allowing for less constipation.

Digestion of Carbohydrates

Monosaccharides do not require breakdown by enzymes, but disaccharides and polysaccharides must be reduced to monosaccharides by enzymes before they can be absorbed and used by the body. Polysaccharides are broken down to disaccharides and disaccharides are broken down to monosaccharides. The splitting of molecules begins in the mouth when polysaccharides mix with salivary amylase and are reduced to disaccharides. Further degradation happens when the reduced molecules come in contact with stomach acids. Disaccharides are passed into the small intestine, where pancreatic amylase completes the breakdown to monosaccharides. These small monosaccharides then pass through the small intestinal villi into the bloodstream, where they travel to the liver for nutrient processing before being sent out to all parts of the body for use as energy.

Box 2-8 indicates enzyme breakdown of disaccharides.

BOX 2.8

- Sucrose is broken down by sucrase into glucose and fructose.
- Maltose is broken down by maltase into glucose units.
- Lactose is broken down by lactase into glucose and galactose.

Problems Associated with Carbohydrates

- Lactose intolerance

    Lactose intolerance occurs when there is an absence of the digestive enzyme lactase. Without lactase, the disaccharide lactose can't be digested or absorbed. It passes undigested to the colon, where bacteria feed on the carbohydrate, resulting in cramping and diarrhea. People who are lactose intolerant must avoid dairy products or take lactase enzyme pills before consuming dairy products. Box 2-10 explains how lactose-intolerant people can get their daily requirement of calcium.

    Certain ethnic groups are at higher risk for lactose intolerance:

    1. Asians

    2. Native Americans

    3. African Americans

- Excessive fiber intake can decrease mineral absorption and cause cramping and gas. Be sure to increase fiber in the diet gradually and drink plenty of water.

- Causes dental caries—simple sugars are most cariogenic (See Chapter 9, Diet and Dental Caries, for more information.)

- Excess consumption of simple CHO can cause a temporary elevation in blood triglycerides, which can increase risk for heart disease.

- Simple sugar load can cause blood glucose to spike and then drop below normal, causing "rebound" hypoglycemia.

BOX 2.9

Lactose-intolerant people can substitute fruit juices fortified with highly absorbable calcium citrate, or take calcium supplements to supply the body with the daily requirement of calcium.

Recommended Daily Intake

There is no recommended daily intake for carbohydrates, but it has been loosely recommended at 55% to 65% of total daily calorie intake, with 25 g to 35 g being fiber. This amounts to about 300 g for a sedentary person and 500 g for a physically active person. It has also been suggested that we limit daily intake of refined sugar to less than 20% of total calorie intake, which includes the sugar present in processed foods like jams, jellies, baked goods, and beverages.

Sugar as a Preservative

Sugar is present in a wide array of processed foods, for example, cereal, canned food products, candy, and baked foods. Like salt, it can be used as a natural preservative, because it pulls water from cells and disables bacteria. Most of the time, its taste is undetectable, as in canned goods, crackers, and processed foods.

Blood Glucose Levels

Normal blood glucose is 80 to 100 mg/dL of blood. When blood glucose is higher, you have *hyperglycemia* (*over*). When blood glucose is lower, you have *hypoglycemia* (*under*).

Maintenance of Blood Glucose Homeostasis

Insulin and **glucagon** are the two hormones involved in maintaining blood glucose levels. When the body has too much blood glucose, we feel an excess of energy and are nervous and excitable. When there is not enough blood glucose, we can feel lethargic, disoriented, and confused. Maintaining the right amount of glucose in the blood is called homeostasis. When the amount of glucose in our blood is in balance with what our body needs, we have an overall sense of well-being and feel just the right amount of energy and alertness. Table sugar and foods rich in simple sugars will overdose our system with glucose, giving us the feeling of both extremes in a short period of time. This is called "spiking" (loading our bodies with sugar) and is a harmful pattern. We feel a rapid surge of energy and a rapid decline in energy in a short time span. When we feel the drop in energy, the first inclination is to eat a candy bar or drink a soda to feel energetic again. This behavior greatly increases the amount of calories ingested (with no nutrients) and lends itself to detrimental long-term effects such as obesity and dental caries. Homeostasis works as follows (and is illustrated in Figure 2-5):

1. Receptor cells in the pancreas recognize that there is more glucose in the blood than the body currently needs for energy. The pancreas secretes the hormone **insulin**, which draws out the excess glucose, reducing the amount of blood glucose when the level gets too high. It attracts glucose from the bloodstream and stores it in the muscle and the liver, where it is converted to glycogen. The glycogen stays in the muscle until the body needs it for energy to move the muscle, and then it is stored in the liver for future energy use. There is a limit to the capacity of glycogen storing cells:

- Once the stores are filled, the overflow is routed to fat.
- Fat cells enlarge and fill with fat.
- Fat cell storage capacity is unlimited.

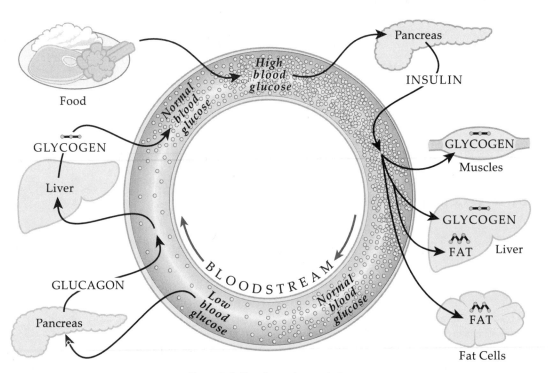

Figure 2-5. Blood sugar homeostasis.

2. Receptor cells in the pancreas recognize that the body is in need of energy so the pancreas secretes the hormone **glucagon**, which converts the glycogen in the liver to glucose and releases it into the bloodstream, where it is carried through the body and used for fuel.

How the Body Regulates Blood Sugar

- Eating carbohydrates throughout the day will help maintain blood glucose levels (see Figure 2-6). Eat a little with each meal.
- Whenever possible, choose the whole grain version of the food, because it is metabolized more slowly by the body.
- Avoid refined sugars—they're empty calories.
- Glycogen that was present in the animal's tissues is depleted when the animal is fasted or frightened before slaughter.

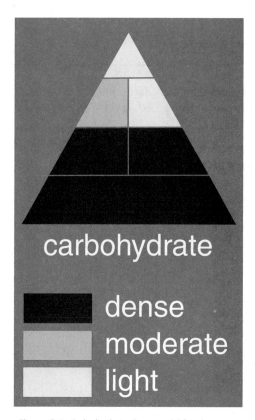

Figure 2-6. Carbohydrates in pyramid food groups.

Counseling Your Patient

If you are providing nutritional counseling for a patient and his or her diet diary reveals a deficiency in the food groups that supply the most carbohydrates (breads and cereals; fruits and vegetables), encourage him or her to eat complex carbohydrates instead of simple carbohydrates. Some patients have difficulty making sudden switches or find that the more fibrous versions of bread, rice, etc., are less palatable. Suggest that they try mixing the simple and complex carbohydrates and gradually increase the proportion of complex carbohydrates until they are able to make the change completely.

For example, you can suggest that patients:

- Mix a few tablespoons of brown rice with white rice.
- Mix whole wheat pasta with semolina pasta.
- When preparing a sandwich, use one piece of white and one piece of whole grain bread, putting the white bread tongue side. Try the same with hamburger buns, rolls, and crackers.
- To increase the servings of fruits and vegetables, drink juice instead of soda.

PUTTING THIS INTO PRACTICE

Your patient has rampant facial caries on her six maxillary anterior teeth. She states that she has a problem staying awake for her job as a bank security guard on the night shift. To stay alert, she drinks a soda every other hour.

1. Would you consider the soda to be a simple sugar or a complex carbohydrate?
2. Give an explanation of what is happening in your patient's body to cause the cycle of low and high energy.
3. Suggest a drink substitution that would give her blood sugar homeostasis.
4. Evaluate your food and drink consumption over the past 2 days and determine if your intake of simple sugars was less than 20% of the total calories in your diet.
5. What changes can you make to better maintain your blood sugar level?

CHAPTER QUIZ

1. Refined sugar would be considered which type of carbohydrate?
   a. Monosaccharide
   b. Simple sugar
   c. Polysaccharide
   d. Complex carbohydrate

2. Which carbohydrate is not absorbed by the body and used as fuel?
   a. Lactose
   b. Sucrose
   c. Glucose
   d. Fiber

3. Insoluble fiber is the type that gives bulk to stools and carries cholesterol out of the body.
   a. True
   b. False

4. Carbohydrates are an excellent low-fat source of fiber and nutrients.
   a. True
   b. False

5. The molecular structure of a complex carbohydrate consists of how many monosaccharides?
   a. At least 2
   b. 4 or more
   c. 10 to 20
   d. Over 100

6. The primary role of carbohydrates in the body is to
   a. provide energy
   b. spare protein
   c. burn fat for fuel
   d. provide the brain with fuel during rest

7. A diet high in carbohydrates will increase a person's chance of developing diseases such as diabetes.
   a. True
   b. False

8. Most digestion of carbohydrates takes place in which body organ?

    a. Mouth

    b. Stomach

    c. Liver

    d. Small intestine

    e. Colon

9. What is the daily recommended intake of fiber?

    a. 50 g to 100 g

    b. 55 g to 65 g

    c. 20 g

    d. 25 g to 35 g

10. Which of the following are the two hormones involved in maintaining blood glucose levels?

    a. Amylase and amylopectin

    b. Insulin and glucagon

    c. Glucose and glycogen

    d. Galactose and fructose

Web Resources

American Society for Nutritional Sciences: Current and Archived Editions of *Journal of Nutrition*
http://www.nutrition.org

Consumer Fact Sheet: Sugar in Your Diet
http://www.sbreb.org/brochures/Fact Sheet/

Current Knowledge of the Effects of Sugar Intake
http://www.ussugar.com/sugarnews/industry/health_effects.html

Tufts Nutrition Navigator: A Rating Guide to Nutrition Websites
http://navigator.tufts.edu/general

Suggested Readings

Davis JR, Stegeman CA. The Dental Hygienist's Guide to Nutritional Care. Philadelphia: W. B. Saunders, 1998.

DuPuy N, Mermel VL. Focus on Nutrition. St. Louis, MO: Mosby, 1995.

Ehrlich A. Nutrition and Dental Health. 2nd Ed. Albany, NY: Delmar, 1995.

Johnson R, Frary C. Choose beverages and foods to moderate your intake of sugars: the 2000 Dietary Guidelines for Americans—what's all the fuss about? American Society for Nutritional Sciences Special Supplement, Symposium: Carbohydrates—Friend or Foe.

Katch FI, Katch VL, McArdle WD. Introduction to Nutrition, Exercise, and Health. 4th Ed. Baltimore: Lippincott Williams and Wilkins, 1993.

Logothetis DD. High Yield Facts of Dental Hygiene. Upper Saddle River, NJ: Prentice Hall, 2003.

Morris WC, Knight EL. Nutrition for Dental Hygienists. Lakeland, FL: ISC Wellness Series, 1993.

Palmer CA. Diet and Nutrition in Oral Health. Upper Saddle River, NJ: Prentice Hall, 2003.

Simin L, Willett WC, Manson JE, Hu FB, Rosner B, Colditz G. Relation between changes in intakes of dietary fiber and grain products and changes in weight and development of obesity among middle-aged women. Am J Clin Nutr. 2003;78 (5):920–927.

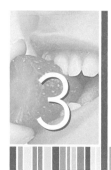

PROTEIN

The Body Builder

Introduction

Proteins, carbohydrates, and lipids are *similar* in that they are composed of the elements carbon, hydrogen, and oxygen, but protein is *different* in that it has the added element of **nitrogen.** Unlike carbohydrates and lipids, protein is not identifiable as a single molecule but is made up of several **amino acids.** Nitrogen is part of the amino acid "building blocks" of protein. There can be thousands of arrangements of amino acids making protein, with each arrangement doing something different for the body. The major function of protein in the body is for GMR: growth, maintenance, and repair (see Box 3-1).

Figure 3-1 illustrates how nitrogen ends up in our food and is outlined below:

- Nitrogen is constantly cycling through the earth's ecosystem and is absorbed from the air into the soil.
- Plants absorb nitrogen from the soil and make amino acids by combining nitrogen absorbed from the ground with carbon fragments produced during photosynthesis.
- Plants link amino acids together to form plant proteins.
- Animals consume plant proteins, which convert to animal protein.
- Animal waste returns nitrogen to the soil.
- Humans consume plant proteins directly or indirectly when we eat animal products.

BOX 3.1

FUNCTION OF PROTEIN

- Growth
- Maintenance
- Repair

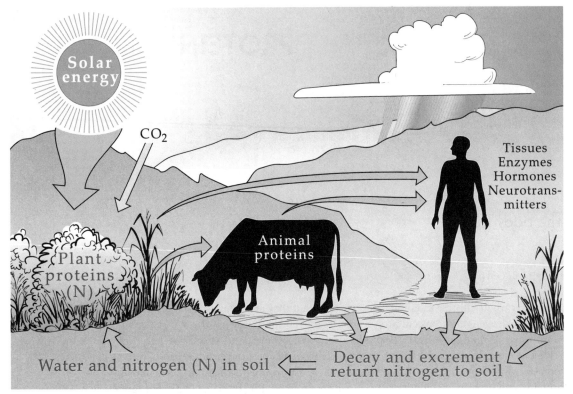

Figure 3-1. The nitrogen cycle.

Box 3-2 lists the components of protein.

Amino Acids

Amino acids are the building blocks of protein. They are made up of:

1. One **organic acid** called a carboxyl group—one carbon atom, two oxygen atoms, and one hydrogen atom: COOH.

BOX 3.2

COMPOSITION OF PROTEIN

- Carbon
- Hydrogen
- Oxygen
- Nitrogen

TEN ESSENTIAL AMINO ACIDS

Phenylalanine   Methionine
Tryptophan   Threonine
Valine   Lysine
Leucine   Arginine
Isoleucine   Histidine

2. One **amino radical**—one nitrogen atom and two hydrogen atoms: NH$_2$

3. Side chains, which can have a combination of carbon and hydrogen atoms.

The side chains are what determine the specific amino acids.

A protein molecule is usually more than 100 amino acids linked together. A **peptide bond** joins amino acids. When two peptide bonds are joined together it is called a *dipeptide bond*; when three are linked it is called a *tripeptide bond*. When there are several hundred peptide bonds linked together, they form a *polypeptide bond*. They can form a string (structural protein) or a three-dimensional shape (functional protein).

Arrangement

Box 3-3 identifies 10 essential amino acids.

Try making different arrangements with these amino acids and you will see that the possibilities are almost endless. Your cells form **nonessential** amino acids from nitrogen and a carbon chain or from a similar essential acid. **Essential** amino acids must be provided through the diet because the body is not able to produce them.

Protein provides the body with many structural and functional processes. The shape of the amino acid determines how the body uses it (see Figure 3-2).

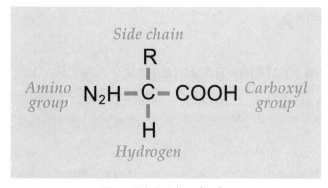

Figure 3-2. Protein molecule.

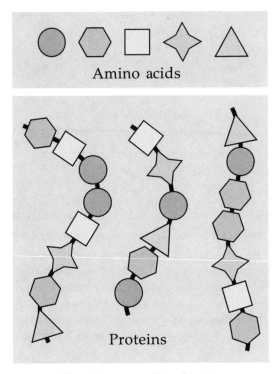

Figure 3-3. Amino acid configuration.

Structural Proteins (Growth)

The body uses amino acid strands to make the following structural parts:

- Skin
- Tendons
- Bone matrix
- Cartilage
- Connective tissue

Functional Proteins (Maintenance and Repair)

Some proteins remain invisible and dissolve in body fluids. The amino acid chains twist and fold into a globular or functional protein (see Figure 3-3) and do the following in the body:

- Regulate activity within the body's fluid compartments.
- Form hormones, enzymes, antibodies, transport proteins (lipoproteins), and chemical messengers (neurotransmitters).

BOX 3.4

MAJOR FOOD SOURCES OF PROTEIN

Animal Sources
- Meat
- Milk
- Eggs
- Fish
- Crustaceans

Sources of Protein

The dairy and meat groups provide the best source of protein. Animal-derived proteins provide the best array of essential amino acids and add a natural salty flavor to meals.

Plant-derived proteins are lower in fat and digest less completely but more quickly than animal sources.

Boxes 3-4 and 3-5 identify animal and plant protein sources.

BOX 3.5

MAJOR FOOD SOURCES OF PROTEIN

Plant Sources
- Legumes
- Peas
- Beans
- Grains

Nutrient Intake Standards

The recommended daily intake (RDI) of protein is estimated to be 40 g to 65 g/day. The amount is calculated as 0.8 g of protein/kg of body weight per day. Example:

weight of 120 lb = 55 kg
$0.8 \times 55 = 44$ g
The RDI of protein for a person weighing 120 pounds is 44 g/day.

Box 3-6 will help you calculate your daily need for protein.

BOX 3.6

CALCULATE YOUR DAILY PROTEIN NEED

_____pounds ÷ 2.2 = _____kg

_____kg × .8 = _____g of protein/day

The amount of protein a person needs is also determined by how much protein they lose each day in urine, feces, sweat, mucus, lost hair and nails, and sloughed skin cells.

Persons under high levels of physical or emotional stress may require more protein. Growth is the major metabolic function of protein during youth, with children requiring more than adults, and maintenance is the primary function after maturity. If a diet contains more protein than the daily requirement, the body has two choices in what to do with any excess: use it for energy or store it as fat.

Protein Quantity and Quality

Protein quantity is measured as nitrogen in the diet. It is ideal for the body to be in nitrogen balance, a measure of how much nitrogen is in the body at the present time. Certain situations will cause the body to be in either *positive nitrogen* balance or *negative nitrogen balance*, both of which should be temporary conditions.

Positive nitrogen balance occurs when there is more nitrogen being absorbed and accumulated in the body than going out. Negative nitrogen balance occurs when there is more nitrogen going out of the body than staying in, signifying loss of body protein. Box 3-7 gives examples of nitrogen entering and exiting the body. Boxes 3-8 and 3-9 indicate situations that cause positive and negative nitrogen balance.

BOX 3.7

Nitrogen balance: The amount of N entering the body is equal to the amount the cells needed to replace parts.

- Nitrogen in = food
- Nitrogen out = urea, feces, sweat, mucus, sloughed skin, lost hair, lost nails

BOX 3.8

POSITIVE NITROGEN BALANCE

Process occurs during periods of growth, pregnancy, muscle building, and repair of tissue after injury.

BOX 3.9

NEGATIVE NITROGEN BALANCE

Process occurs during rapid weight loss, illness, fever, starvation, prolonged metabolic or emotional stress, and protein deficient diets.

BOX 3.10

PROTEIN QUALITY

- Complete
- Incomplete
- Complementary
- Supplementary

Protein quality is determined by how much of each essential amino acid the food contains. Box 3-10 lists examples of protein quality; an explanation is below:

Complete proteins contain all the essential amino acids in the needed proportions. Animal protein provides complete proteins; plant protein provides incomplete protein.

Incomplete proteins are low in one or more of the essential amino acids.

Complementary proteins form an amino acid pattern equal to that found in a complete protein by combining two foods in the same meal. An example would be combining grains and legumes; eaten together, they form a complete protein.

Supplementary protein is a small amount of a high-quality protein added to a meal that is otherwise marginal in terms of protein quantity. An example would be to add cheese or milk to a high-carbohydrate meal.

It was once thought that for the body to utilize complementary or supplemental protein, both had to be consumed together in the same meal. Research has since revealed that the body can utilize foods that have been eaten within a few hours of each other to form complete proteins.

Digestion of Proteins

Digestion of proteins begins in the stomach, where enzymes and acids take apart the protein molecules. As with carbohydrates and lipids, amino acids are absorbed through the small intestinal villi cells and are carried by the blood to the liver. Liver cells use amino acids for protein synthesis or remove the amine group to use the carbon chain for fuel. The liver controls the ratio of the 20 amino acids in the bloodstream.

Protein Deficiency

Protein deficiency symptoms are seen in tissues that are replaced most often—red blood cells and cells lining the digestive tract. Changes that occur in the body because of protein deficiency are as follows:

- Anemia
- Lowered resistance to infection

- Edema
- Brittle and slow-growing hair and nails
- Scaly appearance to skin, with sores that will not heal

Our American diet supplies more than enough protein so deficiencies are rare, but they are still documented in developing countries. The two most documented deficiencies are:

1. Kwashiorkor—lack of dietary protein; edema accounts for the pot-bellied look on starving kids in undeveloped countries.

2. Marasmus—near or total starvation from lack of calories, as in anorexia nervosa.

Protein Excess

How many times have you driven by a restaurant marquee advertising "all you can eat" or a "16-oz steak" on special? In America, our diets tend to have excess protein, sometimes to a gross extreme. What happens when the body ingests more protein than it requires?

- Cells rapidly dismantle excess protein.
- Nitrogen is excreted in urine and remaining carbon is used for energy.
- If the energy supply exceeds demand, the excess carbons are synthesized into fat and stored in adipose tissue.
- Too much excess protein causes kidney and heart disease.

Protein Supplements

Body builders are the number one group supporting sales of protein supplements. Protein is needed for building and maintaining muscles or repairing them from heavy workouts. But our bodies also need protein to make hormones, antibodies, and red blood cells to boost our immune system and to keep our hair, nails, and skin healthy. We can't drink a protein supplement and tell our bodies to make or enlarge muscle mass. Our bodies will take the amino acids and put them together to build the tissue our bodies need most. Whatever is left gets excreted. Most people, including body builders, get enough protein through their diet and do not require protein supplements. Athletes' protein needs will vary depending on whether they are growing, building muscle, dieting, or training for competition. Their protein needs are higher, because the recommended allowance is based on the needs of people who do not exercise. The amino acids are usually used for energy during intense exercise, especially in the absence of carbohydrates. Box 3-11 provides some information on amino acid supplements.

BOX 3.11   AMINO ACID SUPPLEMENTS

Are a waste of money.
The human body needs high-quality protein, not individual amino acids.

Processed and Grilled Meat Health Concerns

Salt and nitrates are used to cure and preserve meat (lunchmeat, ham, bacon, hot dogs, salami, etc.), and both have detrimental effects on health. Excessive salt can have a direct relationship on increased incidence of high blood pressure, and nitrates used to cure meat are converted into cancer, causing nitrosamines in the stomach. For these reasons, it is wise to limit processed meat in the diet. Including foods rich in vitamin C, such as tomatoes and orange juice, with the meal can prevent the conversion of nitrates to nitrosamines.

When using a cooking method with muscle meat, poultry, or fish that results in charring or blackening (e.g., barbecuing or grilling), fat drips onto the coals, forming a smoke that penetrates the meat. The effect of smoke penetrating the meat forms heterocyclic amines and polycyclic aromatic hydrocarbons—both of which are cancer-causing chemicals. It is recommended that lean cuts of meat be used when grilling and to limit foods prepared this way.

Vegetarianism

Many famous people were vegetarians: Socrates, Leonardo da Vinci, Benjamin Franklin, Mahatma Gandhi, Albert Einstein, and Clara Barton, just to name a few. The American Institute for Cancer Research has recently reported that close to 40% of teens identify themselves as vegetarians, and it is estimated that close to 5 million Americans have elected to eliminate meat, poultry, and fish from their diets. Reasons for choosing this eating pattern are varied and include health, religion, ethics, weight, fashion, and environment. The American Dietetic Association has published a new food guide that outlines how to choose a meatless diet but still consume all the needed nutrients. Diets rich in vegetables, fruits, leafy greens, whole grains, nuts and seeds, and legumes can meet the protein needs of people from all age groups and all walks of life.

When meat is excluded from a diet, it leaves room for more carbohydrates, and oftentimes plant sources of protein are forgotten. The type of carbohydrates substituted matters, because eating more simple sugars opens the door for increased chances of caries and diseases. Vegetarians should choose foods wisely and include complex carbohydrates to ensure there is enough protein in the diet. Protein is needed in very small quantities, approximately one out of every 10 calories. In the United States, vegan diets are usually lower in protein than the standard diet; however, the recommendations are very generous and diets high in protein do not appear to have any health advantages. There are several types of vegetarians, depending on what they include in their diets.

These types are described below:

- Lacto-ovo vegetarian—includes eggs and dairy products with meals
- Lactovegetarian—dairy products are only foods of animal origin
- Vegan—consumes no foods of animal origin
- Fruitarian—eats only fruits

 BOX 3.12 Which type of vegetarian would have the least trouble obtaining protein in his or her diet?

Meatless foods that can serve as good protein sources are:

- Beans
- Nuts
- Seeds
- Tofu
- Soy foods
- Vegetarian meat substitutes
- Eggs
- Dairy products

Completely eliminating animal protein from the diet can create a deficiency in one nutrient, *vitamin B-12*, which is found only in animal foods. Lacto-ovo vegetarians need not worry, because B-12 is supplied in cow's milk. A true vegan, however, must supplement his or her diet with fortified soy milk or meat replacement. The deficiency develops over time, affecting the central nervous system, and is not manifested until after the body's stores are depleted, usually 4 years' worth. Once the deficiency manifests, it is irreversible.

Disadvantages of Vegetarianism

Lack of animal foods can cause deficiencies in:

- vitamin B-12
- vitamin D (need exposure to the sun)
- iron (plant iron is not as absorbable as animal iron)
- calcium and riboflavin (can be obtained in soy products)

Meeting calcium needs can be accomplished by including soy milk, soy nuts, fortified fruit juices, fortified cereal, and calcium-rich vegetables such as broccoli, kale, and bok choy. Spinach is also high in calcium, but the oxalate binds with the calcium, reducing its absorption. Box 3-13 lists several advantages to a vegetarian diet.

BOX 3.13

ADVANTAGES OF VEGETARIANISM

Plant proteins are
- Higher in fiber than meats
- Richer in certain vitamins and minerals
- Lower in fat

Benefits of Vegetarianism

- Usually maintain desired weight for height
- Lower blood cholesterol
- Lower rates of some forms of cancer
- Better digestive function
- Benefits the earth

Box 3-14 provides thought for ecological advantages of vegetarianism.

BOX 3.14

ECOLOGICAL THOUGHT

It takes 17 acres of grazing land to produce 1 million calories of animal protein, but one well-developed acre of plants can raise 1 million calories of plant-based protein.

Counseling Your Patient

Most people report more than adequate servings for the meat group because of its abundance in our American diet (Figure 3-4).

If your client reports more servings than suggested for this food group, advise as to what constitutes a serving size. Many people are unaware that restaurant serving sizes are grossly oversized. If the patient is deficient in the meat group, the following suggestions can be made:

- Hard-boil eggs and store them in the refrigerator to add to salads and sandwiches.
- Include cheese, eggs, nuts, and beans with salads.
- Cook a 12-oz steak for dinner, but save half for a sandwich or casserole the next day.
- Include more poultry and fish and less red or fatty meat.
- Educate as to sources of alternative protein—milk, beans, cheese, nuts, etc.

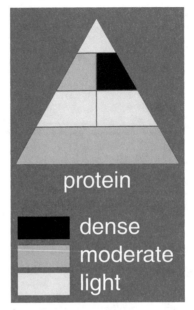

Figure 3-4. Pyramid food groups rich in protein.

- If your client is eating hot dogs or other processed meats, remind him or her to consume them with vitamin C to offset harmful effects of nitrosamines.
- Suggest two meatless dinners each week.
- Encourage meal preparation using chopped chicken, turkey, or beef with pasta or rice, versus large servings of each.

PUTTING THIS INTO PRACTICE

Your patient is a 19-year-old college student who has made the decision to eliminate animal food products from her diet.

1. Write your explanation of the dangers of substituting carbohydrate-rich foods for the calories lost from eliminating protein-rich foods.
2. Calculate her daily protein needs based on a body weight of 126 pounds.
3. List foods that can be included in her diet to ensure an adequate daily protein intake.
4. Write your explanation of how inadequate protein intake can affect the oral cavity.

CHAPTER QUIZ

1. Positive nitrogen balance is when output exceeds input.
    a. True
    b. False
2. Negative nitrogen balance results when a person:
    a. Is pregnant
    b. Is growing
    c. Has a fever or infection
    d. Exercises
3. The role of protein in food is to:
    a. Provide the body with the protein molecule
    b. Supply amino acids so the body can make protein
    c. Provide the body with energy
    d. Build muscle mass
4. A complementary protein:
    a. Contains sufficient amounts of essential amino acids for normal metabolic functions
    b. Contains sufficient quantities of one or more essential amino acids
    c. Is incomplete when ingested singly, but when combined provides all essential amino acids
5. A high-protein diet is hazardous to persons with _____ problems because they retain nitrogen.
    a. stomach
    b. kidney
    c. heart
    d. intestinal
6. Failure of a child to grow because of insufficient protein intake is called:
    a. Marasmus
    b. Protein starvation
    c. Kwashiorkor
    d. Forced malnutrition
7. What are the building blocks of protein?
    a. Amino acids
    b. Linoleic acids
    c. Polyunsaturated fats
    d. Lipoproteins
    e. b and d

8. Lacto-ovo vegetarians omit meat, fish, and poultry from their diets, but include:
   a. All fruits and vegetables
   b. Eggs
   c. Dairy products
   d. All of the above

Web Resources

Atkins Diet and Low Carbohydrate Support (Canada) http://www.lowcarb.ca/

Atkins Nutritionals http://atkins.com/

Beyond Vegetarianism—Transcending Outdated Dogmas http://www.beyondveg.com/

International Vegetarian Union http://www.ivu.org/

The Linus Pauling Institute—Nitrosamines and Cancer http://lpi.oregonstate.edu/f-w00/nitrosamine.html

MedlinePlus Medical Encyclopedia—Protein in Diet http://www.nlm.nih.gov/medlineplus/ency/article/002467.htm

Newswise—Safer Outdoor Grilling Guidelines, Reducing Cancer Risk http://www.newswise.com/articles/view/?id=GRILL.OHM

Purdue University Animal Sciences—Meat Quality and Safety/Reduce Your Cancer Risk From Grilled Meat http://ag.ansc.purdue.edu/meat_quality/grilling.html

The Vegetarian Resource Group http://www.vrg.org/

Suggested Readings

American Dietetic Association, Dietitians of Canada. Position of the American Dietetic Association and Dietitians of Canada: vegetarian diets. J Am Diet Assoc. 2003;103(6):748–765.

Clark N. The power of protein. Physician and Sportsmed. 1996;24(4):11.

Davis JR, Stegeman CA. The Dental Hygienist's Guide to Nutritional Care. Philadelphia: W. B. Saunders, 1998.

DuPuy N, Mermel VL. Focus on Nutrition. St. Louis, MO: Mosby, 1995.

Ehrlich A. Nutrition and Dental Health. 2nd Ed. Albany, NY: Delmar, 1995.

Katch FI, Katch VL, McArdle WD. Introduction to Nutrition, Exercise, and Health. 4th Ed. Baltimore: Lippincott Williams and Wilkins, 1993.

Liebman B. The truth about the Atkins diet. Nutr Action 2002;29:3–7.

Logothetis DD. High Yield Facts of Dental Hygiene. Upper Saddle River, NJ: Prentice Hall, 2003

Mangels R. Protein in the vegan diet. Available at: The Vegetarian Resource Group, http://www.vrg.org/. Accessed June 2003.

Morris WC, Knight EL. Nutrition for Dental Hygienists. Lakeland, FL: ISC Wellness Series, 1993.

Palmer CA. Diet and Nutrition in Oral Health. Upper Saddle River, NJ: Prentice Hall, 2003.

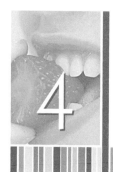

LIPIDS

The Body's Cushion

Introduction

Years ago, being obese signified that a person had enough money to afford the luxury of a steady diet. Today, obesity is considered a harmful epidemic and detrimental to a body's health. An excess of total calorie intake and lipids in the diet can lead to obesity; however, fat, when consumed in moderation, has value in both the diet and body.

Value of Fats

Fats:

- Insulate against the cold
- Cushion organs against injury
- Are components of every body cell
- Are a good source of energy
- Give a sense of satiety and slow digestion
- Carry fat-soluble vitamins A, D, E, and K
- Make food taste good and give it a preferred smooth and creamy texture

The broad category of "lipid" includes oil and fat. As a general rule, lipids are insoluble, which means they do not mix with water; to witness this, try mixing cooking oil or a pat of butter in a glass of water. Box 4-1 identifies the categories of lipids.

Triglycerides

Triglycerides are the largest category of lipid, comprising 95% of all fats found in food and body tissue (body fat = *adipose tissue*). Most triglycerides found in the body are

THREE CATEGORIES OF LIPIDS

Triglycerides
Phospholipids
Sterols

stored as fat. Triglycerides stored in adipose tissue form the body's largest fuel reserve and provide vital insulation. Having fat stored in adipose cells is like having your own utility company to draw from during an energy crisis. Adipose tissue acts as a blanket, insulating the body from the cold, and as a shock absorber, cushioning delicate organs—most notable the kidneys.

Triglyceride molecules contain carbon, oxygen, and hydrogen atoms arranged in two parts: the foundation molecule is *glycerol* and there are three *fatty acid* chains off the side. The fatty acid chains consist of carbon atoms with attached hydrogen and oxygen (COOH) (see Figure 4-1).

Fatty Acids

Triglycerides differ in their fatty acid composition, the difference being the number of carbon atoms in their chains and the number of double bonds. Fatty acid carbon chains can be short, medium, or long:

- Short—less than 6 carbons (short chains mix better in water—like milk)
- Medium—6 to 10 carbons
- Long—more than 12 carbons

Saturation of Fatty Acids

Fatty acids can be categorized as saturated, monounsaturated, or polyunsaturated, depending on how the carbon atoms are bonded together and whether they have a single or double bond. Single bonds between carbons result in a straight flexible chain that

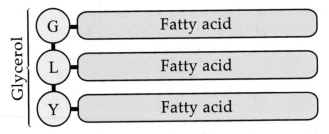

Figure 4-1. Fatty acid.

will pack into a hard fat, like lard, butter, and stick margarine. Think of toy blocks stacking neatly.

The more double bonds a fatty acid has, the softer the fat is at room temperature. Double bonds between carbons result in a bend at the site of the double bond. This bend does not allow the lipid to pack neatly, so it stays liquid at room temperature, like cooking oil. Think of several random toys thrown into a bag, unable to stack together.

The saturation of fatty acids breaks down as follows, which is also illustrated in Figure 4-2:

- Saturated fatty acids (SFAs)—no double bonds
- Monounsaturated fatty acids (MUFAs)—one double bond
- Polyunsaturated fatty acids (PUFAs)—more than one double bond

Source of Lipids

If the source of the lipid is plants, it is considered monounsaturated or polyunsaturated and will be liquid at room temperature, such as olive, corn, and canola oils.

If the source of the lipid is considered a "tropical oil," it is saturated, such as coconut and palm oils. This type is used mainly in cooking.

If the source of the lipid is from animals, it is considered a saturated fat and will be solid at room temperature, such as the marbling of fat in a piece of beef or pork (see Box 4-2). Examples of the different types of fatty acids are presented in Figure 4-3.

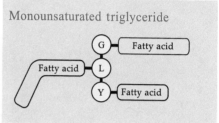

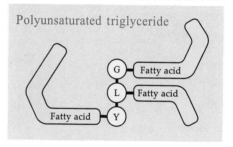

Figure 4-2. Triglyceride bond.

Saturated Fatty Acid

Carbon chains that hold the full number of hydrogen atoms are said to be saturated. A saturated fatty acid tends to raise blood cholesterol levels.

Saturated fatty acids are positively correlated with:

- increased risk of cardiovascular disease
- hypertension
- colon cancer

BOX 4.2

GENERALLY SPEAKING:

- Plant fats are unsaturated and liquid.
- Animal fats are saturated and solid.

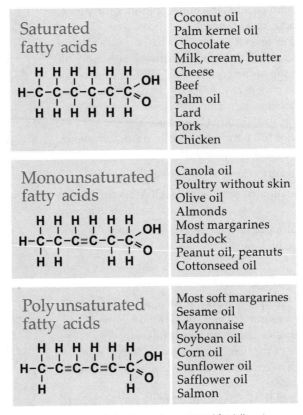

Figure 4-3. Saturated and unsaturated fats/oils.

Unsaturated Fatty Acid

Carbons that hold less than the maximum number of hydrogen atoms will double bond with themselves. (Carbon bonds with another carbon.) Two common unsaturated fatty acids are:

1. monounsaturated (oleic acid)
2. polyunsaturated (linoleic acid)

A *mono*unsaturated fatty acid has one set of the double carbon bonds. Monounsaturated fatty acids have not been associated with any health problems.[1] It is even thought that they may reduce the risk of cardiovascular disease by lowering LDL cholesterol, the harmful cholesterol, and raising HDL, the good cholesterol.

*Poly*unsaturated fatty acids have two or more double carbon bonds. Although polyunsaturated fatty acids have not been directly correlated with health problems, studies are ongoing as to their relationship with certain reproductive organ cancers.

Oxidation of Fatty Acids

Oxygen atoms attach at the point where carbon would attach to hydrogen, which causes the oil to smell and taste rancid. Because fatty acids have nowhere for the oxygen to attach, they are less likely to become spoiled. By adding hydrogen to the place where oxygen can attach to carbons, the oil becomes more resistant to oxygenation, making it more solid at room temperature. This process is called **hydrogenation**.

Hydrogenation

Hydrogenation is a process that infuses hydrogen into the fatty acid chain so that any "vacant" double bonds become full. This type of lipid is called a **trans fat** and affects the body in the same way a saturated fat does.

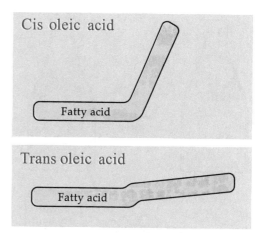

Figure 4-4. Cis and trans fats "kinks."

Food manufacturers use this process to make their product more spreadable, for example, changing corn oil into margarine or making oily natural peanut butter more creamy. Hydrogenation is what turns liquid oil into Crisco or stick margarines. Trans fats make oil more stable so that it can be reused (e.g., for deep frying).

Trans Fat

Most unsaturated fatty acids have the hydrogen atom on the same side of the double bond. This is called the *cis-form*. In the *trans-form*, the hydrogen atoms are on opposite sides of the double bond. This different configuration of the trans-form causes the fatty acid to have a "kink." Figure 4-4 shows the difference between cis and trans oleic acids.

Trans fats are created when oils are "partially hydrogenated." They aren't saturated, monounsaturated, or polyunsaturated. Although trans fats are invisible on the food label, they can build up and be very visible in your arteries. Trans fats raise blood cholesterol as much as saturated fat, making it a secret killer.[2–4]

You can cut trans fats from your diet by:

- avoiding foods listing "partially hydrogenated oil" as an ingredient
- avoiding deep fried foods
- using olive oil or canola oil when cooking
- using margarine from a tub rather than from a stick

Box 4-3 offers an exercise in finding trans fats.

BOX 4.3

READ THE LABEL

Look in your cupboards and pantry and read ingredients listed on the packages of some of your favorite foods. If an ingredient is "partially hydrogenated," then it is a trans fat and affects your body the same as saturated fat.

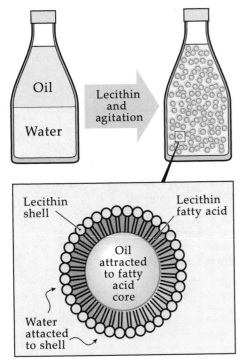

Figure 4-5. Action of a phospholipid.

Essential Fatty Acid

Essential fatty acids are obtained from the food we eat because our bodies can't make them. The two essential fatty acids are omega oils:

1. Omega-3: linolenic acid; found in flaxseed, canola, or soybean oil, walnuts, tuna, and salmon

2. Omega-6: linoleic acid; found in vegetable oils

Omega oil indicates placement of the double bond at the very end of the chain in an unsaturated fatty acid. Omega-3 has been referred to as the anticardiovascular disease nutrient. Because our bodies are always forming and destroying tiny blood clots, the body uses Omega-3 to make substances that reduce blood clot formation, thereby keeping our blood "thin."

Phospholipids

Chemically, phospholipids look like a triglyceride with a phosphorus-containing molecule attached in place of one of the fatty acids. They have the ability to *emulsify*—to hold together molecules of fat and water. Phospholipids are used in cooking and baking to keep ingredients from separating.

A common phospholipid is lecithin (see Figure 4-5), which is found naturally in soybeans and egg yolks.

Read the labels of food in your pantry as suggested in Box 4-4.

Sterols

Sterols are lipids whose carbons form rings instead of chains and contain no fatty acids. Cholesterol is the most common sterol, and its benefit in our diet continues to be debated. Excessive intake of cholesterol-rich foods has been associated with the development of cardiovascular disease, because it promotes build-up of fatty deposits on arteries in genetically sensitive people. Most foods high in cholesterol are also high in saturated fats (see Figure 4-6), which are more detrimental to the arteries than the cholesterol.

BOX 4.4

READ THE LABEL

Check the package of your favorite baked good. Is lecithin listed as an ingredient?

Lipoproteins

Because oil and water don't mix, the body has its own way of allowing fat to travel through the bloodstream to bring lipids to every body cell. Lipoproteins are soluble in both oil and water, so they can circulate freely through the blood. Packaged this way, fats can remain soluble and not separate from liquid blood. Lipoproteins are triglycerides coated with protein, cholesterol, and phospholipids. A **chylomicron** is a type of packaged lipoprotein that is formed during lipid absorption in the small intestines and transported by the lymph system into the bloodstream to be utilized by the body for energy (see Figure 4-7). Those fatty acids not used for fuel are repackaged and stored in adipose tissues.

There are two types of lipoproteins: high-density lipoproteins (HDLs) and low-density lipoproteins (LDLs). HDLs are made in the liver and small intestine and consist of more protein than cholesterol. LDLs , on the other hand, are denser in fat than protein.

LDLs carry the cholesterol to the heart's arteries, where it penetrates the vessel walls, narrows or "clogs" the arteries, and restricts blood flow, giving LDL its unhealthy reputation. HDLs are considered healthy because they actually have a protective factor against LDL. HDLs can remove cholesterol from vessel walls and take it back to the liver, where it is excreted with body waste.

Box 4-5 contains helpful suggestions for remembering the difference between HDL and LDL.

Desirable blood cholesterol should be below 200 mg/dL. An average-weight person should limit daily dietary cholesterol intake to under 300 mg/day.

Table 4-1 indicates the amount of cholesterol contained in certain foods, and Box 4-6 outlines cholesterol guidelines.

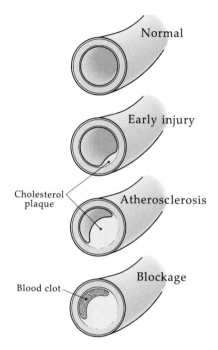

Figure 4-6. Stages of blocked arteries.

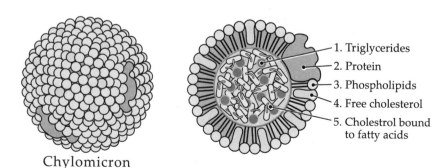

1. Triglycerides
2. Protein
3. Phospholipids
4. Free cholesterol
5. Cholestrol bound to fatty acids

Chylomicron

Figure 4-7. Chylomicron.

↑ LDL = ↑ risk of cardiovascular disease
↑ HDL = ↓ risk of cardiovascular disease

Think of the H in **HDL** and put it in **H**ealthy

Table 4-1. Foods that Contain Cholesterol

1 Cup Food	Mg Cholesterol
Ice Cream	84
Egg noodles	50
Whole milk	34
Low-fat milk	20
Skim milk	5
Chicken liver	800
Beef brains	2,100
Other	
Hot dog	100
Lobster (3 oz)	100
Shrimp (3 oz)	100
Cheesecake (9 in)	2,053

(Taken from Nutrition for Dental Hygienists by Morris and Knight.)

Digestion of Fats

Fats begin their digestion in the stomach with the help of lingual lipase secreted from oral salivary glands and gastric lipase secreted from the stomach. The digestion continues in the small intestine, where chyme (a mixture of food, acids, and enzymes) is emulsified by bile and further broken down by pancreatic lipase. The mixture of reduced fat and bile is absorbed through the small intestinal villi, and the bile returns to the liver. Short-chain and medium-chain fatty acids make their way to the liver, and the long-

CHOLESTEROL GUIDELINES FOR THE AVERAGE AMERICAN ADULT

- LDL level should be less than 130.
- Total cholesterol level should be less than 200.
- HDL levels should be 50–75 or higher.

DIET DEFICIENCY OF LIPIDS

BOX
4.7

- Very rare
- Major symptom is flaky dermatitis

chain fatty acids are converted into a chylomicron and dumped into the lymph system, which carries the chylomicron to the bloodstream.

Recommended Dietary Allowance

It has been suggested that no more than 30% of total calories should be from fat. But it is wise to cut down further because of cardiovascular disease, cancer, weight control, and autoimmune diseases such as multiple sclerosis.[4,5–8]

Boxes 4-7 and 4-8 discuss lipid diet deficiency and excess.

DIET EXCESS

BOX
4.8

- Very common in the United States
- Intake over 30% total calorie intake

Fat in Our Foods

Beware! Fat hides in foods. Removing or trimming fat from meats and poultry will not eliminate significant amounts of cholesterol, and it can eliminate valuable fat-soluble vitamins. Decreasing dietary fat is not the final answer to lowering blood cholesterol, because the liver can make cholesterol from saturated fat. Box 4-9 contains an acronym to help you choose meat products.

FIRST

BOX
4.9

Choose your meat products according to this acronym

F = Flank
R = Round
S = Sirloin
T = Tenderloin

Environmental Concerns

Plants and animals absorb fat-soluble chemicals, such as pesticides, that are stored in fat and oil. People who use these plants and animals as food will absorb some of the stored chemicals, such as dichlorodiphenyltrichloroethane (DDT).

Major Reasons to Reduce Dietary Fat:

- Reducing dietary fat decreases the risk of cardiac disease, the number one killer of Americans over the age of 40.
- High-fat diets are associated with increased risk of cancer.[5]
- The number of obese children has doubled in the last 25 years.[9]

Counseling Your Patient

When analyzing a patient's diet diary, consider if his or her food choices are high fat or low fat. Sections of the Food Pyramid that contain the most lipids are the dairy and meat group (see Figure 4-8).

Eighty-five to ninety percent of the calories in cheese come from fat, much of which is saturated. Patients can choose almost any food from the fruit and vegetable food group, because they are almost fat-free. Three exceptions are olives, avocados, and coconuts.

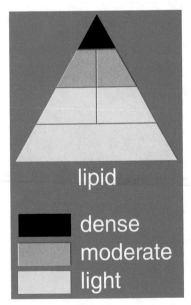

lipid

dense

moderate

light

Figure 4-8. Pyramid food groups rich in lipids.

- If your patient is drinking whole milk, a sudden switch to skim or fat-free milk may be too big of a change and result in failure. Suggest gradually switching by drinking 2% for a few weeks, then switching to 1% for a few weeks, and then eventually working down to fat-free. Sometimes mixing the two—whole and skim—works also. There is just as much calcium in skim milk as there is in whole milk.
- If your patient is using high-fat spreads, suggest trying some of the fat-free margarines and cream cheeses.
- When choosing a topping for baked potatoes and in pasta salads, fat-free salad dressings and salsa are good substitutions.
- Encourage using monounsaturated and polyunsaturated cooking oils.
- Educate about trans fats and teach your client how to spot them on food labels.

Your patient is a 250 lb male who lumbers back to the operatory.

He has difficulty fitting in the treatment chair and is clearly out of breath from the mild exertion of walking and sitting. He makes the comment that he has to "lose some weight" and asks if you have any advice.

Keeping in mind that it is not within the realm of dental nutritional counseling to "put a patient on a diet," think about some words of wisdom you can offer this patient.

1. List diseases that are caused by excess lipid consumption.

2. How can your patient find out if a food product contains a trans fat?

3. If your patient doesn't want to give up the amount of food he eats, give him examples of low-fat foods that can replace high-fat foods.

4. Would you expect to see any oral changes from the consumption of foods with excess fat?

CHAPTER QUIZ

1. Which lipid, when consumed in excess, causes the most disease to the human body?
    a. Saturated fat
    b. Unsaturated fat
    c. Polyunsaturated fat

2. Which of the following examples of lipids would have the most double bonds?
    a. Butter
    b. Margarine
    c. Lard
    d. Olive oil

3. Eliminating foods high in cholesterol from the daily diet will reduce a person's total cholesterol level.
    a. True
    b. False

4. Hydrogenating corn oil does not change the fact that it is a monounsaturated fatty acid.
    a. True
    b. False

5. It is recommended that the number of calories obtained from fat in our daily diets be less than 10%.
    a. True
    b. False

6. The largest category of lipid in the body is:
    a. Phospholipids
    b. Sterol
    c. Triglycerides
    d. Chylomicron

7. The specialized molecule that is soluble in both lipid and water is called:
    a. Triglyceride
    b. HDL
    c. Lipoprotein
    d. Omega-3

8. Which of the following are functions of lipids in the body?
    a. Maintain blood glucose level and provide energy
    b. Manufacture hormones and enzymes
    c. Repair and build new tissue
    d. Cushion organs and insulate against the cold

9. Triglycerides found in animal fat are composed mainly of what type of fatty acid?
   a. Monounsaturated
   b. Disaturated
   c. Polyunsaturated
   d. Saturated

10. The fatty acid that is low in LDL and high in HDL and is good for serum cholesterol is called:
    a. Fully saturated
    b. Monounsaturated
    c. Polyunsaturated
    d. Omega-3

Web Resources

All About Lowering Cholesterol http://www.all-about-lowering-cholesterol.com/high-cholesterol-foods.html

Eating to Lower Your High Blood Cholesterol http://www.medhelp.org/lib/step.htm

References

1. Lada AT, Rudel LL. Dietary monounsaturated versus polyunsaturated fatty acids: which is really better for protection from coronary heart disease. Curr Opin Lipidol. 2003;14(1):41–46.

2. Food and Drug Administration, HHS. Food labeling: trans fatty acids in nutrition labeling, nutrient content claims, and health claims. Final rule. Fed Regist. 2003;68(133):41433–41506.

3. Steinhart H, Rickert R, Winkler K. Trans fatty acids: analysis, occurrence, intake and clinical relevance. Eur J Med Res. 2003;8(8):358–362.

4. Clifton PM, Keogh JB, Noakes M. Trans fatty acids in adipose tissue and the food supply are associated with myocardial infarction. J Nutr. 2004;134(4):874–879.

5. Liebman, B. Fat chance—extra pounds can increase your cancer risk. Nutr Action 2003;30(8):3–8.

6. Lichtenstein AH, Kennedy E, Barrier P, Danford D, Ernst ND, Grundy SM, Leveille GA, Van Horn L, Williams CL, Booth SL. Dietary fat consumption and health. Nutr Rev. 1998;56(5, pt 2):S3–19.

7. Lichtenstein AH. Dietary fat and cardiovascular disease risk: quantity or quality? J Womens' Health 2003;12(2):109–114.

8. Hu FB, Willett WC. Optimal diets for prevention of coronary heart disease. JAMA 2002;288(20):2569–2578.

9. Nicklas T, Johnson R. Position of the American Dietetic Association: dietary guidance for healthy children ages 2 to 11 years. J Am Diet Assoc. 2004;104(4):660–677.

Suggested Readings

Davis JR, Stegeman CA. The Dental Hygienist's Guide to Nutritional Care. Philadelphia: W. B. Saunders, 1998.

DuPuy N, Mermel VL. Focus on Nutrition. St. Louis, MO: Mosby, 1995.

Ehrlich A. Nutrition and Dental Health. 2nd Ed. Albany, NY: Delmar, 1995.

Grundy SM. The optimal ratio of fat-to-carbohydrate in the diet. Annu Rev Nutr. 1999;19:325–341.

Katch FI, Katch VL, McArdle WD. Introduction to Nutrition, Exercise, and Health. 4th Ed. Baltimore, Lippincott Williams & Wilkins, 1993.

Logothetis DD. High Yield Facts of Dental Hygiene. Upper Saddle River, NJ: Prentice Hall, 2003.

Morris WC, Knight EL. Nutrition for Dental Hygienists. Lakeland, FL: ISC Wellness Series, 1993.

Palmer CA. Diet and Nutrition in Oral Health. Upper Saddle River, NJ: Prentice Hall, 2003.

Rao AV. Lycopene, tomatoes, and the prevention of coronary heart disease. Exp Biol Med. 2002;227(10):908–913.

Renaud S, Lanzmann-Petithory D. Coronary heart disease: dietary links and pathogenesis. Public Health Nutr. 2001;4 (2B):459–474.

Sanders TA. Olive oil and the Mediterranean diet. Int J Vitam Nutr Res. 2001;71(3):179–184.

Schaefer EJ. Lipoproteins, nutrition, and heart disease. Am J Clin Nutr. 2002;75(2):191–212.

Tande DL, Hotchkiss L, Cotugna N. The associations between blood lipids and the Food Guide Pyramid: findings from the Third National Health and Nutrition Examination Survey. Prev Med. 2004;38(4):452–457.

Wolfram G. Dietary fatty acids and coronary heart disease. Eur J Med Res. 2003;8(8):321–324.

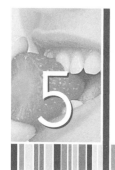

VITAMINS

Directors of Cell Processes

Introduction

"Vitamine" was the term coined by Casimir Funk (1884–1967) for the unidentified substances present in food that prevented the diseases scurvy, beriberi, and pellagra.[1]

Vitamins are calorie-free molecules needed by the body in very small quantities to help with metabolic processes. They are essential, which means they must come from outside the body, supplied in the food we eat or as a dietary supplement. A common misconception is that "vitamins give you energy." The truth is, vitamins *help* with the metabolic reaction that releases energy within the food molecules, making them the directors of cell processes. But if the body has an adequate supply of vitamins to help with the creation of energy, taking more will not make you more energetic.

Vitamin discovery, both accidental and deliberate, was spread out over 40 years. By 1940, all 13 currently recognized vitamins had been discovered and given a sequential letter of the alphabet. With the discovery and medicinal use of vitamins, thousands of people were cured of debilitating and fatal diseases. Although it is true that vitamins will cure diseases, the specific deficiency must first be present for the vitamin to work its magic. Box 5-1 itemizes properties of vitamins.

BOX 5.1

WHAT ARE VITAMINS?

- Molecules
- Essential
- Organic
- Noncaloric
- Needed in small amounts for cellular metabolism

Table 5-1.	Properties of Vitamins

Vitamin	Name
A	Retinol
B-1	Thiamin
B-2	Riboflavin
B-3	Niacin
B-6	Pyroxidine
B-9	Folate
B-12	Cobalamine
H	Biotin
C	Ascorbic Acid
D	Calciferol
E	Tocopherol
K	Koagulations

Categories of Vitamins

Vitamins have alphabet/numeric and common names. Table 5-1 identifies both.

Vitamins are also divided into one of two solvent categories: fat soluble or water soluble. Water-soluble vitamins include vitamin C and all the B vitamins. Fat-soluble vitamins are A, D, E, and K. Figure 5-1 identifies water- and fat-soluble vitamins.

Whether the vitamin is fat- or water-soluble depends on:

- which foods supply the vitamin
- vulnerability of the vitamin during cooking
- how the vitamin functions in the body
- whether the body can store the vitamin

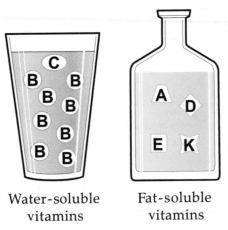

Water-soluble
vitamins

Fat-soluble
vitamins

Figure 5-1. Fat-soluble and water-soluble vitamins.

Daily Recommended Intake

Only minute amounts of any one vitamin are required on a daily basis. Vitamin C has the highest daily requirement of approximately 60 mg. To give you an idea of how much this is: One teaspoon is equivalent to 5,000 mg. It would take $2^1/_2$ months worth of appropriate vitamin C intake to give you one teaspoonful. Vitamins are found in all food groups, with fruits and vegetables being especially rich. Vitamin B-12 is the only vitamin found exclusively in animal food, whereas all other vitamins can be obtained from both plants and animals. (See individual vitamins for specific recommended intakes and food sources.)

Digestion and Absorption

Vitamins are *released* from food during the digestive process but are not *digested*.

Water-soluble vitamins (vitamin B-complex and C) that are utilized by the body for metabolic processes are absorbed through the small intestine. Any excess that is not used right away is excreted by the kidneys in the urine.

Fat-soluble vitamins (vitamins A, D, E, and K) are absorbed with dietary fats through the small intestine. After absorption, they are sent to the liver and fat depots and circulate through the blood with the help of chylomicrons and lipoproteins.

Toxicity/Imbalance

Eating too many fortified foods or taking a megadose of vitamin supplements—more than the recommended daily intake—can produce toxic effects. Fat-soluble vitamins are more toxic than water-soluble vitamins because they can be stored and accumulate in adipose tissues. There is less danger of water-soluble vitamins exerting a toxic effect on the body because storage is limited and usually the excess is excreted on a daily basis.

Vitamin D is the most toxic of all vitamins because of its ultimate effect on the human body. Vitamin D enhances the absorption of calcium, and so an excess of vitamin D causes an excess of calcium circulating in the blood, which is detrimental to the heart.

Two water-soluble vitamins can be somewhat toxic: vitamin B-6 and niacin. Both can have detrimental effects if the amount ingested is more than the kidney can handle and excrete. Box 5-2 lists the most toxic vitamins.

BOX 5.2

TOXICITY

Vitamin D is the most toxic of all vitamins.
Vitamin B-6 is the most toxic *water*-soluble vitamin.

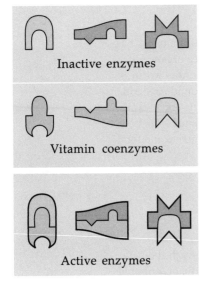

Inactive enzymes

Vitamin coenzymes

Active enzymes

Figure 5-2. Vitamin coenzymes.

An imbalance of vitamins occurs when too much of one vitamin is added to an adequate diet, causing a deficiency of others. The B-complex vitamins function as a group, one no more important than the other. Excess of one of the B vitamins can throw off the biochemical balance, creating a deficiency in its cofactors. Figure 5-2 illustrates how vitamins function as coenzymes.

How the Body Makes Its Own Vitamins

If a diet is *in*sufficient in certain vitamins needed for metabolic processes, the body has the capability to manufacture some, but not all. This is accomplished by the body using existing chemicals to synthesize vitamins that resemble those we consume in food or supplements. The chemical the body draws on is called a *precursor*. Box 5-3 lists examples of vitamins the body manufactures with a precursor. Once the diet remedies the vitamin deficiency, the body will stop producing the vitamin and use what is supplied in food.

The body can also make vitamin K, biotin, and pantothenic acid with the help of resident bacteria in the colon.

Major Functions of Vitamins

Vitamins perform the following functions in the body:

- Energy metabolism: B1 (thiamin), B2 (riboflavin), B3 (niacin), biotin, and pantothenic acid help convert calories released from carbohydrates, lipids, and proteins into energy by producing adenosine triphosphate (ATP). ATP is to the body what gas is to a car.
- Tissue synthesis: Vitamins A, D, B6 (pyroxidine), and C help form body cells—epithelium, bone, and collagen.
- RBC Synthesis: Vitamins B9 (folic acid), B12 (cobalamin), E, and K help bone marrow form new red blood cells (RBCs). The life of an RBC is approximately 4

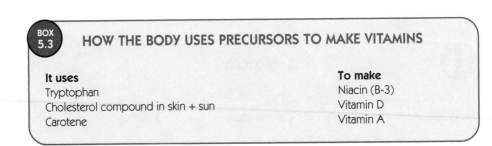

BOX 5.3 HOW THE BODY USES PRECURSORS TO MAKE VITAMINS

It uses	To make
Tryptophan	Niacin (B-3)
Cholesterol compound in skin + sun	Vitamin D
Carotene	Vitamin A

months, so maintenance of an adequate supply demands continual use of body resources. A lack of one or more vitamins at the time of development will manifest as anemia. The type of anemia depends on the vitamin in which the body is deficient.

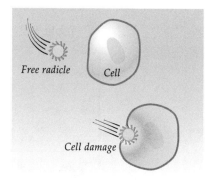

- Antioxidants: Vitamins A, C, and E serve as protectors from damaging free radicals—oxygen atoms in search of other atoms to attract. As a rule, oxygen travels through the body in pairs. When they disengage and become single, they search for other atoms with which to bond. Once an oxygen atom becomes a free radical, a chain reaction occurs, releasing other oxygen atoms to become free radicals, and body cells get damaged in the process. This cell damage has been blamed for causing certain cancers, arteriosclerosis, cataracts, and other aging diseases because of damage to DNA. Vitamins protect the body by making themselves available to intercept the single oxygen atoms before the chain reaction is set off.

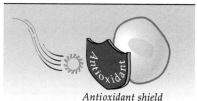

Figure 5-3. Antioxidant action.

Vitamin A in its precursor form, beta-carotene, is the preferred chemical for antioxidant function. It is the orange-yellow pigment enclosed in fibrous cell walls of plants.

Research for antioxidants is ongoing, so it is important to review the literature frequently to give accurate advice to patients. Presently, there is more support *not* to recommend antioxidants because they may not have the desired effect and can be harmful for some people when taken in large doses.[2-4] Figure 5-3 illustrates how antioxidants protect cells.

Other functions of vitamins include boosting the immune system, keeping the mind alert, helping with hormone production, and synthesizing genetic material. Table 5-2 lists vitamins and their specific functions.

Vitamins and Food Processing

To ensure that food remains vitamin-rich after processing, manufacturers may enrich or fortify their products. *Fortification* occurs when vitamins and minerals are added to the food product, such as in cereals and milk with added vitamins A and D. *Enriched* food products add nutrients that were lost during processing to the level present in the unprocessed product, such as flour, rice, and bread.

Food processing submits ingredients to high temperatures, light, and oxygen—all detrimental to water-soluble vitamins. Boiling food on the stovetop causes nutrients to be released from the food into water; to retain these nutrients, this water can be used to cook something else—for example, rice, mashed potatoes, or soup. Prolonged exposure to heat, as in crockpot cooking, roasting, and frying, can actually destroy water-soluble vitamins. Careful consideration of food preparation can preserve vitamins so that they

Table 5-2. Functions of Vitamins

Function	Vitamin
Energy metabolism	Thiamin B-1
	Riboflavin B-2
	Niacin B-3
	Biotin
	Pantothenic Acid
Tissue synthesis	A
	D
	Pyroxidine B-6
	C
RBC synthesis	Folate B-9
	B-12 Cyanocobalamine
	E
	K
Antioxidants	A
	C
	E

can benefit your body when consumed in the food. Stir frying at a high temperature seals in nutrients, and short cooking time reduces nutrient loss. Microwaving uses a small amount of water and high temperature for a short amount of time, also preserving most of the vitamins' properties.

The following are some healthful tips when choosing produce to ensure the maximum benefit from the vitamins provided:

- When selecting fresh foods remember that the shorter the time from vine to table, the more nutrients. Nutrient value diminishes as the produce ages.
- Shop at roadside stands for homegrown produce that has not been sprayed with chemicals to delay ripening.
- If purchasing produce from the frozen food section in a grocery store, shake the bag to be sure it isn't a frozen block of ice. One solid piece in the bag indicates that the product has thawed, which will cause nutrients to leak into the water.
- Canned produce is the least desirable because of the heat used to sterilize it and the added salt and sugar for preserving.

Figure 5-4 illustrates the loss of vitamin C during food preparation.

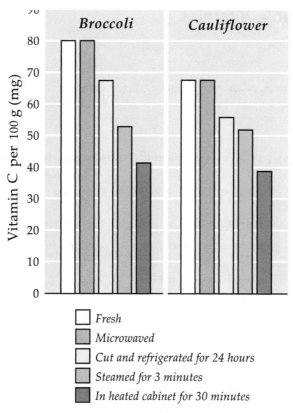

Figure 5-4. Loss of vitamin C during food preparation.

Vitamin Charts and Lists

Most vitamins serve the body in more than one capacity and can be found in multiple foods. Reading charts and lists from textbooks and websites can cause the reader quite a bit of confusion. One source may list a particular vitamin as being involved in blood cell synthesis while another might state that the vitamin is needed for 100 different enzyme actions in protein synthesis. Another may list some foods that contain the vitamin while yet another may list four new ones. It is almost impossible to make a complete and comprehensive vitamin document, so most references glean important facts and try to arrange them in an organized way. For the purpose of this textbook, an attempt has been made to highlight *major* functions, sources, deficiency and excess states, and recommended daily intake (RDI). The list is neither comprehensive nor all encompassing, but it can serve as a resource for initial vitamin inquiry. Vitamin information has been organized into water-soluble and fat-soluble categories.

Water-Soluble Vitamins

Thiamin: B-1

Function

Thiamin functions as a coenzyme in energy metabolism by converting calories released from carbohydrates, lipids, and proteins into energy.

Source

Best source is pork but it is also abundant in fortified cereals and grains, meat, poultry, peanut butter, and eggs.

Deficiency State

Beriberi—symptoms include:

- Loss of appetite, muscle weakness, loss of sensation in the extremities, mental confusion
- Enlarged and irregularly beating heart
- Burning tongue, loss of taste
- Occurs in people who eat large amounts of white rice or flour
- Common in alcoholics

RDI

Our need for thiamin increases as we consume more carbohydrates and expend more energy. Recommended daily intake is approximately 1.1 mg.

Riboflavin: B-2

Function

Riboflavin helps with production of ATP and releasing energy from carbohydrates, lipids, and proteins.

Source

Sources are milk or milk products (yellow-green fluorescent pigment in milk whey), meat, poultry, fish, and enriched and whole grain breads and cereals.

Deficiency State

Ariboflavinosis—symptoms include:

- Tissue inflammation and deterioration
- Angular chelosis: cracks in corners of mouth and lips
- Cracks in skin folds around nose
- Glossitis: atrophy of filiform papillae, swollen, dark red tongue
- Extra blood vessels in cornea with itching, tearing, and sensitivity to light
- Greasy and scaly looking skin

RDI

Requirement for riboflavin depends on total calorie intake, energy needs, body size, and growth rate. Recommended daily intake is around 1.1 mg.

Niacin: B-3

Function

Niacin is needed for all cell functions and is a coenzyme and partner to riboflavin. It also converts glucose released from food to energy and assists with blood cell formation.

Source

Meat is a major food source as well as poultry, fish, dark-green leafy vegetables, enriched breads and grains, peanuts, beans, and peas.

Deficiency State

Pellagra—symptoms include:

- The three D's: dermatitis (skin turns black when exposed to the sun), diarrhea, and dementia
- Also a fourth D: eventual death

Excess State

- Causes facial flushing
- Decreased blood lipids (popular treatment for high cholesterol in the 1980s)
- Can cause liver damage; chronic overdosing can require a liver transplant

RDI

Recommended intake is approximately 14 mg/day.

Pyroxidine: B-6

Function

Pyroxidine functions as coenzyme in reactions for amino acid, fatty acid, and carbohydrate metabolism. It also assists with formation of blood cells. Pyroxidine gained popularity in the 1980s as a cure for premenstrual syndrome (PMS) and carpal tunnel syndrome but is no longer considered helpful to these syndromes.

Source

Best food sources include anything of animal origin—meat, poultry, fish, pork, liver, and eggs—as well as brown rice, whole-wheat, lentils, and peanuts.

Deficiency State

Deficiency states are microcytic anemia, depression, convulsions, depressed immune system, angular chelosis, and glossitis.

Excess State

Vitamin B6 is the most toxic water-soluble vitamin because it can be stored in the muscle and liver. Long-term megadosing may cause permanent neurologic damage that includes numbness in extremities and uncoordinated muscle movement.

RDI

The more protein consumed, the more vitamin B6 the body requires. Its bioavailability is affected by 40 different medications, including isoniazid (treatment for tuberculosis). Recommended intake has been set around 1.4 mg/day.

Folate: B-9 (Folacin, Folic Acid)

Function

Folate synthesizes amino acids, assists with red blood cell maturation, and synthesizes DNA and RNA.

Source

Food sources include fortified breads and grains, yeast, kidney, and dark-green leafy vegetables. Folate was originally extracted from spinach (folium = leaf).

Deficiency State

Deficiency of B9 causes fetal neural tube defects and macrocytic anemia. Deficiencies are often seen in alcoholics and found to cause abnormal GI function—irritability, exhaustion, and loss of appetite.

RDI

Medications can interfere with bioavailability: aspirin, oral contraceptives, anticonvulsants, and some anticancer drugs. Recommended intake is approximately 400 mcg daily.

Cobalamine: B-12

Function

Cobalamine converts folate into the form in which it can be used to produce red blood cells and nucleic acids for DNA synthesis.

Source

Sources are from animal foods only: meat, poultry, fish, eggs, and dairy products.

Deficiency State

Deficiency in B-12 may cause pernicious anemia, also known as macrocytic anemia; this takes about 5 years to manifest. This is rare but can be found in vegans who eat no animal products. It causes permanent brain and nerve damage, resulting in eventual paralysis of extremities.

Excess State

There are no known toxic side effects from excess ingestion, but because of its pretty red color, it is used in research studies as a placebo.

RDI

Recommended intake is approximately 2.4 mcg daily.

Biotin: H

Function

Biotin assists in releasing energy from carbohydrates, lipids, and proteins. It also acts as a coenzyme in the synthesis of RNA and DNA.

Source

Bacteria in intestines assist the body in making biotin. Food sources are liver, yeast, legumes, nuts, and egg yolks.

Deficiency State

Deficiency is rare but causes depression, anorexia, nausea, dark-red swollen tongue, scaly skin, and hair loss. It has been *mistakenly* presumed by some that if a deficiency causes hair loss, then an excess would cause hair growth.

RDI

This vitamin contains sulfur and is needed in tiny amounts, approximately 30 mcg daily.

Pantothenic Acid

Function

Pantothenic acid serves as a coenzyme that assists with the release of energy from carbohydrates, fats, and proteins. It also assists with vitamin D synthesis.

Source

Pantothenic acid is found everywhere (including the sun) and is in almost every food. It can be manufactured in the intestines by bacteria.

Deficiency State

Because this vitamin is in every living thing, deficiencies are rare. If one does exist, symptoms could include burning feet, fatigue, nausea, and poor muscle coordination, and cramping.

RDI

Recommended intake has been set at approximately 5 mg daily.

Vitamin C: Ascorbic Acid

Function

Vitamin C assists with collagen formation, strengthens immune system, aids with iron and calcium absorption, and helps with amino acid metabolism. Vitamin C is a natural antihistamine and can shrink swollen tissues. If sinuses are inflamed during a cold or flu, increasing ingestion of vitamin C offers temporary relief from swollen tissues, which gives it its curative reputation.

Source

Food sources are kiwi, citrus fruits, cantaloupe, strawberries, leafy green vegetables, and cruciferous vegetables.

Deficiency State

Scurvy—symptoms include:

- Anemia, bleeding gums, nosebleeds, poor digestion, easy bruising
- Merchant seafaring vessels packed limes for daily consumption, giving sailors the nickname of "limeys"

Excess State

The eyes, adrenal glands, and brain have the ability to store high concentrations of vitamin C for about 3 months. Because it can be stored, excesses are possible. Symptoms include:

- GI upset
- Diarrhea
- Orange-colored urine
- Interference with anticoagulants
- Iron toxicity

RDI

Smokers need to consume two times the amount to compensate from loss from alterations in metabolism. Recommended intake is approximately 60 mg daily.

Fat-Soluble Vitamins

Vitamin A

Function

Vitamin A assists with formation of epithelium, skin, and mucous membranes. It also maintains healthy eyes and assists with bone remodeling (dismantles existing bone).

Source

Food sources are carrots, yellow and orange fruits and vegetables, spinach and broccoli, liver, eggs, butter, and fortified foods.

Deficiency State

Hypovitaminosis A—symptoms include:

- Dry, bumpy skin, poor immunity, slow growth
- Night blindness, xeropthalmia (total blindness)
- Dry epithelium
- Increased incidence of skin, lung, and bladder cancer

Excess State

- Common because of supplements and fortified foods
- Symptoms are headache, vomiting, double vision, hair loss, bone abnormalities, liver damage

RDI

Recommended intake is approximately 800 mcg/day.

Vitamin D

Function

Vitamin D is really a hormone that facilitates the absorption of calcium and phosphorus and regulates their presence in plasma. It assists with bone formation by aiding the absorption of calcium.

Source

The body has the ability to manufacture from the sun (fair-skinned, 30 minutes; dark-skinned, 3 hours). Food sources are liver, egg yolks, and fish oil.

Deficiency State

Rickets (children) and osteomalacia (adult form of rickets); symptoms of rickets include:

- Pigeon-breasted (prominent sternum) and bow-legged (poorly formed bones)
- Nocturnal elevated body temperature (fever)
- Diffuse body soreness and tenderness
- Slight pallor
- Diarrhea
- Liver and spleen enlargement
- Delayed dentition and poorly calcified teeth

Fortified milk eliminated this problem in the United States, but it is still common worldwide. It is most prevalent in extreme climates that keep people inside or keep them wearing clothing that protects them from the sun.

Excess State

The more vitamin D in the body, the more calcium is absorbed and circulating in the bloodstream. Excess calcium collects in soft tissues and can produce calcium stones in the kidneys. It also causes calcifications or hardening of blood vessels, which can be pathologic to the heart.

Symptoms of excess are:

- Nausea, vomiting, and headaches
- Irreversible damage to kidneys and cardiovascular tissue

RDI

Recommended intake is approximately 5 to 10 mcg daily.

Vitamin E

Function

Vitamin E acts as an antioxidant and protects red blood cells.

Source

Sources are margarine and vegetable shortening, salad dressing, whole grains, nuts, and legumes.

Deficiency State

Deficiency is not common but can manifest as hemolytic anemia that causes breakage of red blood cells.

Excess State

Vitamin E excess symptoms include:

- Nausea
- Diarrhea
- Cramps and bleeding
- Interference with anticoagulant drugs

RDI

Recommended intake is approximately 15 mg daily.

Vitamin K

Function

Vitamin K functions as a cofactor for the synthesis of prothrombin required for blood clotting.

Source

It is manufactured by intestinal bacteria; food sources include dark-green leafy vegetables.

Deficiency State

Deficiency is caused by diseases that reduce fat absorption or by using broad-spectrum medications that kill intestinal bacteria. Symptoms include prolonged bleeding and increased clotting time.

Excess State

High doses of vitamin K can interfere with anticoagulants, which could result in hemorrhaging.

RDI

Recommended intake is approximately 100 mcg/day.

Table 5-3 lists the vitamins and their deficiency states.

As a dental health care provider, it is important to know the oral considerations of vitamin deficiencies. Table 5-4 outlines oral deficiency symptoms.

Table 5-3. Deficiency States of Vitamins

Vitamin	Deficiency
A	Xeropthalmia—night blindness, dry eyes
B-1	Beriberi
B-2	Ariboflavinosis
B-3	Pellagra
B-6	Microcytic anemia—small RBC
B-9	Neural tube defects of fetus
B-12	Pernicious anemia
C	Scurvy
D	Rickets—children Osteomalacia—adults
E	Hemolytic anemia—RBC breakage
K	Hemorrhage—failure of blood to clot

Table 5-4.	Oral Deficiency Symptoms
Vitamin	**Oral Deficiency Symptoms**
A	Xerostomia
	Oral leukoplakia
	Hyperkeratosis
	Hyperplastic gingival tissue
B	Red swollen lips with vertical fissures and chelosis
	Burning, smooth, red tongue, which may be ulcerated, geographic, with atrophied papillae
	Red, ulcerated, burning gingival tissues
C	Red-purplish, swollen, bleeding gums
	Loose teeth
	Slow healing
D	Failure of bone wounds to heal
	Enamel hypocalcification
	Loss of alveolar bone
	Thinning of trabeculation
E	No known deficiency symptoms
K	Failure of wounds to stop bleeding

Counseling Patients

The following tips are taken from the Mayo Clinic website and may be of interest to your patients when discussing vitamins:

- "Supplements are not substitutes." There is no substitute for wholesome foods that supply other nutrients like complex carbohydrates, fiber, and other phytochemicals.
- Synthetic supplements are the same as "natural" vitamins, so there is no need to pay a lot for supplements. The body does not recognize the difference between natural and synthetic vitamins.
- Never take more than 100% of the recommended daily intake of any one vitamin. Megadosing on supplements increases your body's need for that nutrient, and cutting back to the required level may cause a pseudo deficiency. When you increase intake of one vitamin, you need to increase its cofactors.
- Store vitamin supplements in a cool, dry place. Never place or store the container in a hot or humid place such as the bathroom.

BOX 5.4

NATURAL VERSUS MANMADE

The human body cannot distinguish between manmade and naturally produced vitamins.

If the patient has a health problem, always check with a doctor, pharmacist, or registered dietitian first. Some vitamins react negatively with medical conditions. For example, high doses of niacin can harm the liver, vitamins E and K interfere with anticoagulants, men who drink alcohol and take beta carotene have a higher incidence of prostate cancer, and smokers who take beta-carotene have an increased incidence of lung cancer.

BOX 5.5

VITAMIN Q

Recently a team of researchers at the Institute of Physical and Chemical Research in Tokyo published a report claiming that they have isolated PQQ (pyrroloquinoline quinone), with chemical properties similar to vitamin B-6. They believe this discovery is the first new vitamin since 1948 and will include it with vitamins B-2 and B-3, calling it Vitamin Q. Currently, PQQ is not included in multivitamin/mineral supplements, but it can be consumed in the diet with parsley, green peppers, kiwi fruit, papaya, spinach, tofu, tea, and certain meats.

PUTTING THIS INTO PRACTICE

1. Vitamins should dissolve in the stomach within 30 minutes to make them available to the body when they pass to the small intestines. If they do not dissolve with help from hydrochloric acid in the stomach within this time, they can pass through to the intestines whole and will not be available to the body. Cover your vitamin supplement with vinegar, which will determine if it will dissolve in time to be utilized by the body.

2. Compare an inexpensive brand of vitamins to a more expensive brand for vitamin content. Place the labels side by side and determine if the bottles contain the same number and percentage of vitamins.

CHAPTER QUIZ

1. What are the recommended antioxidant supplements?
   a. Vitamin B-complex with C
   b. Vitamins A, D, and E
   c. Vitamins C, E, and A (beta-carotene)
   d. Calcium and vitamins C and E

2. If an adult patient complained of a burning, sore tongue that was very shiny and red when you examined it, which vitamin could you safely assume he was lacking?
   a. Vitamin E
   b. Vitamin C
   c. Vitamin B-2
   d. Vitamin A

3. If the patient you treated on Tuesday morning arrived for treatment Thursday morning and stated that she never stopped bleeding from the scaling and root smoothing, which vitamin could she be lacking?
   a. Vitamin A
   b. Vitamin D
   c. Vitamin E
   d. Vitamin K

4. Which of the following categories of vitamins can be more toxic to the human body?
   a. Water-soluble
   b. Fat-soluble

5. The body absorbs natural vitamins far better than synthetic vitamins.
   a. True
   b. False

6. Which vitamin can be the most toxic if taken in large doses?
   a. Vitamin C
   b. Vitamin A
   c. Vitamin D
   d. Vitamin B-6

7. Scurvy is a deficiency state of which vitamin?
   a. Vitamin A
   b. Vitamin K
   c. Vitamin C
   d. Pyroxidine

8. Which one of the following statements is false of the B-complex vitamins?

   a. They can be lost during food processing

   b. They are water soluble

   c. They act as coenzymes

   d. They are stored in the body's fat depots

9. Excess of one B vitamin can throw off our biochemical balance.

   a. True

   b. False

10. Enriched foods contain added vitamins and minerals, and fortified foods have nutrients added back to their level before processing.

    a. True

    b. False

Web Resources

Center for Disease Control and Prevention—Folic Acid Now, Before You Know You're Pregnant http://www.cdc.gov/ncbddd/fact/folnow.htm

Dispelling Fears of Vitamin D Toxicity http://www.cholecalciferol-council.com/toxicity.pdf

Mayo Clinic—Drugs and Supplements Information http://www.mayoclinic.com/findinformation/druginformation/listinvoke.cfm?range=U-Wz

MedlinePlus Medical Encyclopedia—Vitamins http://www.nlm.nih.gov/medlineplus/ency/article/002399.htm

National Institute of Health—Facts About B6 http://www.cc.nih.gov/ccc/supplements/vitb6.html

National Institute of Health—Facts About Folate http://www.cc.nih.gov/ccc/supplements/folate.html

U.S. Food and Drug Administration—Folic Acid Fortification http://vm.cfsan.fda.gov/~dms/wh-folic.html

References

1. Funk C. The Vitamins. Baltimore, MD: Williams and Wilkins, 1922.

2. Hasnain BI, Mooradian AD. Recent trials of antioxidant therapy: what should we be telling our patients? Cleve Clin J Med. 2004;71(4):327–334.

3. Hlubik P, Sstritecka H. Antioxidants—clinical aspects. Cent Eur J Public Health 2004;12(Suppl):S28–30.

4. Stanner SA, Hughes J, Kelly CNM, Buttriss J. A review of the epidemiological evidence for the "antioxidant hypothesis." Public Health Nutr. 2004;7(3):407–422.

Suggested Readings

Abraham J, Smith HL, eds. Regulation of the Pharmaceutical Industry. London: Palgrave, 2003.

Asimov I. The Chemicals of Life. New York: Abelard-Schuman, 1954.

Combs G. The Vitamins. San Diego, CA: Academic Press, 1992.

Davis JR, Stegeman CA. The Dental Hygienist's Guide to Nutritional Care. Philadelphia: W. B. Saunders, 1998.

DuPuy N, Mermel VL. Focus on Nutrition. St. Louis, MO: Mosby, 1995.

Ehrlich A. Nutrition and Dental Health. 2nd Ed. Albany: Delmar Learning, 1995.

Is Your Supplement Dissolving? Tufts University Health and Nutrition Letter 1977;15(9).

Katch FI, Katch VL, McArdle WD. Introduction to Nutrition, Exercise, and Health. 4th Ed. Baltimore, Lippincott Williams and Wilkins, 1993.

Liebman B. Antioxidants. Nutr Action. April 2002.

Liebman B. Do you know your vitamin ABC's? Nutr Action 1999;26(7).

Logothetis DD. High Yield Facts of Dental Hygiene. Upper Saddle River, NJ: Prentice Hall, 2003.

Morris WC, Knight EL. Nutrition for Dental Hygienists. Lakeland, FL: ISC Wellness Series, 1993.

Palmer CA. Diet and Nutrition in Oral Health. Upper Saddle River, NJ: Prentice Hall, 2003.

Smith R, Olson R, eds. The Biographical Encyclopedia of Scientists. New York: Marshall Cavendish Corporation, 1998.

Touger-Decker R. Oral manifestations of nutrient deficiencies. 1998;65(5/6): 355–361.

Vitamins and minerals: how much is too much? Interview with Robert Russell. Nutr Action 2001;28(5).

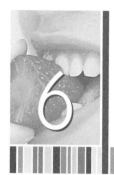

MINERALS

Regulators of Body Fluid

Introduction

Usually when one discusses vitamins, the mention of minerals is not far behind. Because they are combined in dietary supplements, it seems that they are inseparable. Minerals, like vitamins, are essential chemical elements. They are different, however, in that they are metals with electrical charges, not separate molecules; are inorganic (whereas vitamins are organic); and are noncaloric because they do not contain carbon. Many necessary minerals are provided in food and water and are found within our body's water content. We need to replace minerals every day by eating food or drinking water, making use of the minerals we need and excreting those that we don't need. The body must be efficient in balancing minerals because excess of one can cause an imbalance of another, leading to disease. Box 6-1 identifies factors of minerals.

Function of Minerals

As with vitamins, the body needs minerals for many metabolic functions. Making up 4% of the body's mass, minerals are found in hormones and enzymes and assist the body in the following ways:

- For controlling water balance, muscle contraction, and nerve transmission: Sodium, potassium, and chloride control fluid inside and outside our body cells and maintain exchange of nutrients and waste. Fluid compartments are either *intracellular* (within a cell) or *extracellular* (outside the cell wall). Metabolic work takes place inside the cells, and fluid outside the cells transports nutrients and waste throughout the body. Water is constantly passing in and out of cell membranes with the help of electrically charged minerals sodium, potassium, and chloride. This is sometimes referred to as the "pumping action" that maintains homeostasis—water balance—within and between our cells.

WHAT ARE MINERALS?

- Essential
- Inorganic
- Noncaloric
- Metals
- Small electrically charged particles

- For tissue synthesis: Iron, calcium, and magnesium assist with the formation of teeth, bones, and blood. Zinc assists with the synthesis of eye pigment needed for night vision and the formation of collagen tissue.
- For energy metabolism: Phosphorus precipitates energy metabolism and is part of adenosine triphosphate (ADT). It is also part of lipoproteins, which transport lipids in blood.
- As essential cofactors in chemical reactions: Copper and iron work together to aid with the synthesis of hemoglobin.
- As facilitators in the antioxidant process: Selenium and sulfur work in tandem with vitamins A, C, and E, bonding with free oxygen radicals to avoid cell destruction.

Source of Minerals

As with vitamins, there is no best food source that contains all minerals. A varied diet with selections from all food groups, specifically unrefined foods, will ensure an adequate intake. All essential minerals are ingested through our diets—through drinking water and our food choices. Minerals are found in oceans, lakes, and rivers as well as in the soil where our food is grown. They enter the food chain by way of plants absorbing them from the soil and water and animals eating the plant. To complete the cycle, decaying plants and animals return minerals to the soil. The minerals end up on our table in the food we eat and the beverages we drink. Figure 6-1 illustrates the mineral cycle.

Categories of Minerals

There are two categories of minerals: major and trace, depending on body needs. Major minerals are needed in quantities greater than 100 mg/day and trace minerals are needed in quantities less than 100 mg/day. There are six major minerals:

- Calcium
- Chloride
- Magnesium
- Phosphorus

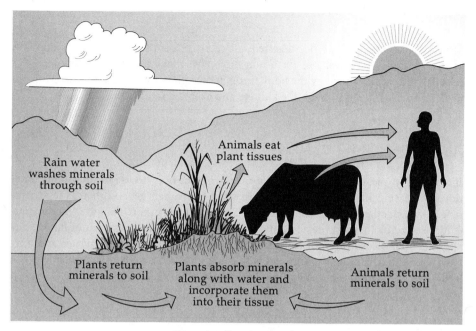

Figure 6-1. The mineral cycle.

- Potassium
- Sodium

Some of the more common trace minerals are:

- Chromium
- Cobalt
- Copper
- Fluoride
- Iodine
- Iron
- Lithium
- Manganese
- Molybdenum
- Nickel
- Selenium
- Sulphur
- Tin
- Zinc

Digestion

Minerals, like vitamins, are not digested but released from foods during the digestive process, making them available for use in the body's many metabolic functions. Once released, they are absorbed by the body through the villi in the small intestine. Minerals not utilized are filtered through the kidneys and excreted in the urine.

Bioavailability

Bioavailability means that a mineral is available for the body to use for metabolic functions. Increasing intake of one mineral can affect how others get absorbed as they compete with each other for bioavailability. For example, taking more than the recommended dose of zinc can affect the absorption of copper, and increasing calcium intake may alter the body's absorption of iron. Also, phytochemicals known as phylates and oxylates, found in certain foods, can bind with minerals and make them unavailable to the body. Box 6-2 identifies minerals affected by these chemicals.

Mineral Ions

If an electron is added or removed from a neutral atom, it forms an ion. Minerals can be either positively charged *cations* (+) or negatively charged *anions* (-). An ionic compound is made of a combination of positive and negative ions. Many dietary minerals appear in the ionic form, switching the "ine" suffix to "ide." Examples are fluorine becoming fluor*ide* and chlorine becoming chlor*ide*. Metal anions team up with cations, forming ionic compounds in food. A good example is sodium and chloride making salt. You may see the minerals named in textbooks as either the element or ion, but for the purpose of this text, they will be referred to as the ion.

Mineral Deficiency

A carefully chosen diet will provide an abundance of all minerals needed for daily metabolism, making supplements unnecessary. Occasionally deficiencies do exist because of diets that restrict or eliminate foods rich in the following minerals: calcium, potassium, iron, zinc, and magnesium. Those who are lactose intolerant (see Chapter 2) may elim-

BOX 6.2   **PHYLATES AND OXYLATES**

- Phylates and oxylates bind with minerals and prevent their absorption.
- Phylates are found in fiber and bind with zinc.
- Oxylates are found in leafy greens and bind with calcium.

inate calcium-rich dairy products from their diets, creating a deficiency in calcium. People with anorexia nervosa, who are on severe calorie-restricted diets, eventually develop a deficiency in potassium. Because of monthly blood loss, many young women are found to be deficient in iron. Strict vegetarians (vegans) who eliminate all forms of animal products and who are not efficient in combining proteins may develop a deficiency in zinc. Severe alcoholics who choose drinking alcohol over eating will develop a deficiency in magnesium over time. A deficiency in each of these minerals will manifest their own set of symptoms. (See specific minerals for a list of deficiency symptoms.) Box 6-3 lists common mineral deficiencies.

BOX 6.3 **COMMON DEFICIENCIES**

- Calcium
- Zinc
- Iron
- Magnesium

Mineral Excess

Processed foods are the bane of our existence. The convenience of packaged, canned, and microwavable food make them a daily staple, but consumers should beware: Processed foods have an abundance of sodium and chloride. Sodium and chloride together make table salt, which is used as a preservative; salt draws fluid out of bacteria, rendering it ineffective. These two minerals are blamed for an increased incidence in hypertension for those who are salt-sensitive. Ingesting an excess of many minerals can have a toxic effect on the body, although potentially toxic minerals are less absorbable than those with a low potential for toxicity.

Minerals That Function as Electrolytes

Osmosis is when fluid passes freely from one side of a permeable membrane to another. The "sodium pump" in the human body works by osmosis, with fluid being equalized on both sides by electrical charges inside and outside cells. Sodium (+) and chloride (-) work together outside the cell wall and potassium (+) works within. Box 6-4 lists minerals that are considered electrolytes.

BOX 6.4 **ELECTROLYTES**

- Sodium
- Potassium
- Chloride

Sodium (Na+)

Function

Sodium is a soft silvery metal that is one of the two elements of table salt. It is used liberally as a food additive for flavoring, as a preservative, and to flavor baking soda. It functions as a cation (positive charge) in *extracellular* fluid to regulate fluid balance.

Sources

Sources include table salt, meat, eggs, dairy products, unprocessed produce and grains, legumes, and most processed foods.

RDI

The recommended daily intake (RDI) would fit in the palm of your hand. The suggested daily minimum, 50 mg, includes sodium added during processing and after preparation; most diets, however, average around 2,000 mg. An intake of $1/4$ teaspoon/day is safe, with an upper intake of no more than $1^1/4$ teaspoon/day.
Figure 6-2 illustrates recommended sodium intake.

Deficiency and Excess

Because of its widespread use in processed food, deficiency is rare and excess more common. Disease of excess is hypertension.

Chloride (Cl–)

Function

Chloride is the partner to sodium in table salt. Together they work in *extracellular* fluid to maintain the body's fluid balance.

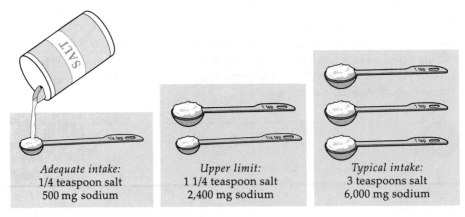

Adequate intake:
1/4 teaspoon salt
500 mg sodium

Upper limit:
1 1/4 teaspoon salt
2,400 mg sodium

Typical intake:
3 teaspoons salt
6,000 mg sodium

Figure 6-2. Recommended sodium intake.

Source

Sources include table salt, meat, fish, eggs, and processed foods.

RDI

Recommended daily consumption is approximately 750 mg.

Deficiency

Deficiency is rare because of its abundance in processed foods.

Potassium (K+)

Function

Potassium is the "man on the inside" found in *intracellular* fluid, working with sodium and chloride on the "outside" in extracellular fluid to maintain water balance in the body's fluid compartments. It plays an essential role in muscle contractions and neurologic transmissions

Source

Potassium is found in meats, grains, fruits and vegetables, and processed foods.

RDI

Recommended daily intake is approximately 2,000 mg.

Deficiency and Excess

Deficiency is rare but can happen during a state of dehydration. The confusion from dehydration prevents one from knowing that a problem exists. Deficiency symptoms are also apparent in those whose diets are severely restricted. Symptoms of deficiency include:

- Nausea and vomiting
- Listlessness
- Muscle cramps
- Cardiac arrest
- Respiratory failure

Excess can cause:

- Numbness of extremities, face, and tongue
- Muscle weakness
- Cardiac arrhythmias: the heart will dilate and quit contracting

Box 6-5 explains the importance of adequate potassium when taking diuretic medication.

BOX 6.5 — DIURETICS

Potassium is lost in the urine when a person is placed on diuretics to help lower blood pressure. Diuretics rid the body of fluid so that less pressure is placed on the vessels, thereby reducing blood pressure. Many patients who are on diuretics are instructed by their physician to eat a banana or drink a glass of orange juice every day to replenish lost potassium.

Minerals for Energy Metabolism

Box 6-6 lists minerals needed for energy metabolism.

BOX 6.6 — MINERALS FOR ENERGY METABOLISM

- Phosphorus
- Magnesium
- Manganese
- Iodine
- Chromium

Phosphorus (P)

Function

Phosphorus assists with the formation of teeth and bones: 80% of the phosphorus in the body is stored in teeth and bones. It also acts as an enzyme in energy metabolism and protein synthesis and is necessary for muscle contractions.

Source

Food sources are anything that is protein-rich: meat, eggs, poultry, fish, legumes, and dairy products.

RDI

Recommended daily intake is around 700 mg.

Deficiency and Excess

Deficiency can happen if a person consumes antacids: Many antacids contain aluminum, which competes with phosphorus for absorption (bioavailability). If aluminum-containing antacids are consumed over a long period of time, changes in bone density, such as osteoporosis and osteomalacia, may occur.

Magnesium (Mg)

Function

Magnesium is a silver-white metallic mineral essential for mineralization of bones and teeth: 60% is stored in bones and teeth, 39% in soft tissues, and 1% in extracellular fluid. It also assists with protein synthesis and neuromuscular activity and is a cofactor in utilization of ATP.

Source

Food sources are green leafy vegetables, nuts, meats, legumes, and grains.

RDI

Recommended daily intake is approximately 400 mg.

Deficiency and Excess

Dieting and gastric bypass surgery can affect the absorption of magnesium, as can drinking "soft" water devoid of the mineral. The body can "sweat out" magnesium during excess exercise and lose it during bouts of chronic diarrhea and alcoholism.[1] Symptoms of a magnesium deficiency include nausea, muscle spasms, hallucinations, and mental derangement. High calcium intake can depress absorption of magnesium (bioavailability competition). Excess can occur from long-term use of antacids listing magnesium as an ingredient.

Manganese (Mn)

Function

Manganese is needed for many enzyme reactions. It also helps metabolize carbohydrates and assists in synthesizing bones of inner ear.

Source

Food sources are plants and grains.

RDI

Recommended daily intake is approximately 2 mg.

Deficiency and Excess

Deficiency in manganese is associated with poor reproduction rates, growth retardation, skeletal abnormalities, and bad balance. Excess has been noted in miners who are environmentally exposed to high levels of manganese and exhibit the following symptoms: Parkinson's disease, speech impairment, headaches, and leg cramps.

Iodide (I)

Function

Iodide is part of the hormone thyroxin that regulates our pace of work and mental development.

Source

Sources of iodide are iodized salt, seawater, and seafood.

RDI

Recommended daily intake is approximately 150 mg.

Deficiency and Excess

A deficiency will manifest as a goiter, which appears as an enlarged thyroid gland. Symptoms would be those related to decreased thyroid hormone function—hypothyroidism: weight gain, dry skin and hair, low blood pressure, intolerance of cold, and lethargy. Figure 6-3 illustrates a goiter.

Myxedema is another deficiency condition that happens when the thyroid gland decreases its absorption of iodine or there is not enough supplied in the diet. It manifests with decreased metabolic rate, slow, slurred speech, enlarged tongue, swollen hands, brittle hair, drowsiness, and increased sensitivity to cold temperatures.

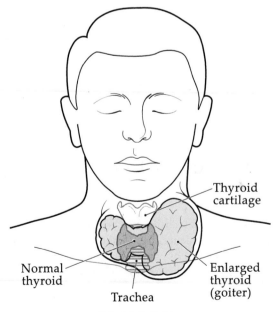

Figure 6-3. Goiter.

Chromium (Cr)

Function

Chromium is essential for glucose and energy metabolism. It is a cofactor in insulin production and needed for uptake of insulin by cell membranes.

Source

In the diet, chromium is found in whole grains, beer, fats and oil, meat, yeast, mushrooms, and prunes.

RDI

Recommended daily intake is about 30 mg.

Deficiency and Excess

Deficiency in chromium may resemble diabetes in that it results in poor glucose tolerance. This is seen more in patients on intravenous feedings.

Minerals Needed for Tissue Synthesis

Box 6-7 lists minerals that help with tissue synthesis.

BOX 6.7

MINERALS NEEDED FOR TISSUE SYNTHESIS

- Calcium
- Fluoride
- Zinc

Calcium (Ca+)

Function

A growing body needs calcium to build healthy teeth and bones. Calcium is the most abundant mineral in the body, with 99% found in teeth and bones. The other 1%, available in blood and soft tissue, is used for conducting nerve signals, contracting muscles, keeping cell membranes permeable, forming bridges between collagen strands, and acting as cofactor in the synthesis of blood-clotting protein. These physiologic needs of calcium are so vital to survival that the body will actually take calcium from bone to support these functions, before it uses it to maintain bones.

Although bones may appear to be hard, static structures, calcium is constantly being removed and replaced. As the body ages, the ability to absorb calcium is diminished. Children can absorb around 75% of the calcium supplied in their diets, whereas adults

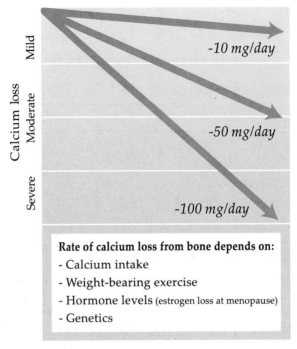

Figure 6-4. Rate of calcium loss.

can absorb only about 25%. In anticipation of this decreased absorption, calcium is stored in bones, creating a "warehouse of calcium," until the age of 35 when absorption and storage ability are reduced. The body has the capability of storing about 10 years' worth of calcium for future bone remodeling and physiologic functions. Figure 6-4 diagrams rate of calcium loss.

Source

Think "Milk—Bones—Stones." Best food sources are dairy products, animal bones such as sardines, stone-ground cornmeal and lime-processed tortillas, tofu, broccoli, and legumes. Orange juice with added calcium is also a very good daily source.

RDI

A 1,200 mg recommended daily intake has been suggested for maintenance of healthy bones and physiologic function.

Deficiency and Excess

If calcium is deficient in the diet during the growth years, the result is reduced bone mineralization. *Osteomalacia* means "soft bones." When this occurs in children it is called

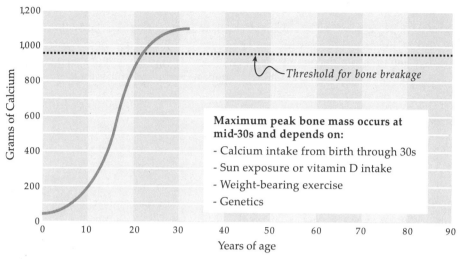

Figure 6-5. Threshold for bone breakage.

rickets, which is the deficiency disease of vitamin D. Because vitamin D assists the body in absorbing calcium, the two are symbiotic. (See Chapter 5 for vitamin D deficiency state.)

Osteoporosis is a disease where there is not enough calcium to maintain bone, resulting in a net loss of structure. The importance of storing calcium in the teen years should be emphasized to reduce the risk of osteoporosis and bone fractures. The disease proceeds faster in women after menopause because of the decrease in estrogen production.[2,3] Weight-bearing activity puts stress on bones, helping them retain calcium and decreasing resorption.

Figure 6-5 illustrates the threshold for bone breakage. Figure 6-6 illustrates osteoporosis.

It was once believed that calcium supplements increased the incidence of kidney stones. Recent studies have shown that normal calcium intake with supplementation does not contribute to this risk.[4–6]

Fluoride (F)

Fluoride is the only mineral that is considered nonessential. We do not need to include it in our diet for important physiologic functions.

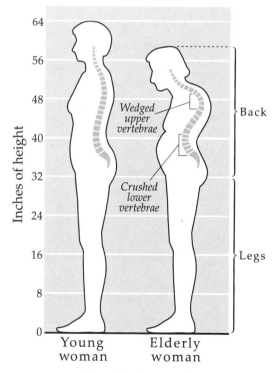

Figure 6-6. Osteoporosis.

Function

Fluoride increases retention of calcium in teeth and bones. If consumed by the pregnant woman or infant, it becomes incorporated into the developing tooth structure. The hydroxyl ion in the tooth combines with the fluoride ion to form fluorohydroxyapatite, which makes the structure less soluble and more resistant to demineralization.

Source

Fluoride is found in drinking water, soil, tea, and seafood.

RDI

Because fluoride is nonessential, there is no recommended daily intake; however, a daily intake of approximately 3 mg can prevent defective enamel development.

Deficiency and Excess

A fluoride deficiency correlates with increased incidence of dental caries. An excess of fluoride during tooth development can manifest as dental fluorosis: This appears clinically as mottled enamel or enamel hypoplasia, which is incomplete development of tooth enamel due to inadequate calcium and phosphate metabolism.[7-10]

Zinc (Zn)

Function

Zinc assists in protein metabolism, synthesizing DNA during cell division, and development of pigment needed for night vision; it aids in immune response and with insulin storage in the pancreas. Zinc is also involved in taste and smell sensitivity and helps with wound healing. In addition, it serves as a cofactor in over 200 enzyme systems.

Source

Meat, poultry, and fish offer more bioavailable zinc than plant sources.

RDI

Recommended daily intake is about 10 mg.

Deficiency and Excess

A deficiency in zinc can cause anorexia (loss of appetite), slow tissue repair, night blindness, mental lethargy, and a loss of taste and smell.

An excess of zinc can interfere with copper absorption, alter cholesterol metabolism, and weaken blood vessels. Toxicity can occur in people who eat food cooked in galvanized pots and pans.

Minerals Needed for Red Blood Cell Synthesis

Box 6-8 lists minerals that synthesize red blood cells.

 BOX 6.8 **MINERALS NEEDED FOR RED BLOOD CELL SYNTHESIS**

- Iron
- Copper

Iron (Fe)

Function

About 20% of the iron in the body is stored in bone marrow, the liver, and the spleen to act as a reserve in times of iron depletion. The rest of the iron in the body can be found in the blood. The iron in hemoglobin binds with oxygen in the lungs and carries it to other cells in the body, where it is exchanged for carbon dioxide.

Source

The source of iron in the diet makes a difference in its bioavailability. More iron is absorbed from animals (40%) than plants (10%). Iron from animal sources is called *heme* iron and from plant sources is called *nonheme*.

- Heme iron food sources include meat, fish, and poultry.
- Nonheme iron is found in egg yolks, leafy greens, and legumes.

Vitamin C helps with absorption of iron. Drinking orange juice or including other foods rich in vitamin C can enhance the uptake of iron from the meal.

RDI

Recommended daily intake is 8 mg for men and 18 mg for women.

Deficiency and Excess

Iron is usually well-conserved in the body because the kidneys will not excrete it. Iron stores can be depleted during bleeding from any cause—including menstruation, bleeding ulcer, or extreme wound. Females can lose up to 45 mg of iron during menstruation. This along with a poor diet accounts for up to 50% of American women exhibiting iron deficiencies. Iron deficiency anemia is one of the most prevalent world nutritional problems.

Anemia is detected through a blood test that shows hemoglobin levels less than needed to supply the oxygen demands of the body. There will be a decrease in the number of red blood cells and low plasma levels. Symptoms of anemia are:

- Pallor
- Angular cheilosis

- Lethargy
- Apathy
- Short attention span
- Irritability

Iron is the most toxic mineral because the body has the capacity to store it. Excess absorption occurs with overconsumption of vitamin C.

Hemochromatosis is a hereditary disease where there is increased iron absorption from the small intestines.[11]

Copper (Cu)

Function

Copper aids the absorption of iron and with iron, works to synthesize hemoglobin. Copper is also needed for regulating blood lipid levels and assists with collagen formation and nerve function.

Source

Food sources include liver, whole grains, nuts, legumes, vegetables, fruit, water from copper water pipes, and chocolate cooked in copper pots.

RDI

The recommended daily intake is approximately 1.5 mg.

Deficiency and Excess

Deficiencies are rare but can happen with excess intake of zinc, because these two minerals compete for bioavailability.

Antioxidants

Box 6-9 lists minerals that assist in the antioxidant process.

BOX 6.9

ANTIOXIDANTS

- Selenium
- Sulfur

Selenium (Se)

Function

Selenium is a trace mineral that works with vitamin E as an antioxidant.

Source

Food sources depend on the abundance of selenium in soil and animals that eat plants grown in the soil. Because of this it is geographically higher in some areas than others. Foods containing selenium are grains, vegetables, and meats.

RDI

Recommended daily intake is approximately 60 mcg.

Deficiency and Excess

A selenium deficiency can cause cardiac weakness. An excess can cause hair loss, fatigue, and vomiting.

Sulfur (S)

Function

Sulfur is part of the vitamins biotin and thiamin. It is also found in enzymes that are part of the body's drug-detoxifying pathway. Sulfur is needed for liver function and also to maintain the acid-base balance of body fluid.

Source

Food sources include meat, poultry, fish, and legumes; it is also found in food preservatives.

RDI

There is no recommended daily intake for sulfur.

Deficiency and Excess

There are no known deficiency or toxicity states.

Nonnutritive Mineral Ingestion

Lead and mercury are two minerals that are highly toxic. Although their addition to one's diet is not intentional, they enter the body inadvertently by ingestion or absorption through the skin.

Lead (Pb)

Lead is a soft blue-gray metallic element that is used to make batteries, solder seals, wheel weights, TV tubes, foil or wire, x-ray shields, soundproofing material, and ammunition. It is very toxic and can be ingested by drinking water that flows through lead-soldered water pipes or by consuming food prepared in lead cookware and lead crystal. It can also be inhaled from household dust and air or pass through the skin from soil or hair dye.

Two commercial products, paint and gasoline, included lead in their ingredients but have since reconfigured their formulas, thereby reducing the incidence of lead poisoning. The greatest source of lead poisoning is still from deteriorating paint used in residential housing before 1978. Paint formulas prior to this date included lead, which gave the paint a sweet taste and made it desirable for children to eat chipped paint. Until recently, lead in gasoline controlled the "knocking" in engines. Inhaling exhaust fumes or the air around busy highways contributed to many cases of lead poisoning. Effects of lead poisoning include: reduced IQ, learning disabilities, stunted growth, impaired hearing, memory and concentration problems, fertility problems, and nerve disorders.

Mercury (Hg)

Mercury, also called quicksilver, is a shiny metallic liquid that beads up and can be made to roll around. It is not required for any metabolic functions. Mercury is found naturally in the environment and is released into the atmosphere through industrial pollution. Particles fall through the air into bodies of water, where it turns into methylmercury. Fish living in rivers and streams absorb methylmercury, which can then be consumed by humans. Although the human body can tolerate small amounts of mercury, it can be a health concern for certain groups of people. Nervous systems of infants, growing fetuses, and young children with small body mass can be harmed by ingesting too much methylmercury. Fish and shellfish, with their omega-3 fatty acids and high protein content, have many healthful benefits and shouldn't be completely eliminated from the diet. The U.S. Department of Health and Human Services has suggested eating smaller and younger fish to eliminate mercury and choosing more fish from the low-mercury category.

- Fish with high levels of mercury are shark, swordfish, king mackerel, or tilefish.
- Fish low in mercury are shrimp, canned tuna (albacore has more mercury than canned light tuna), salmon, pollock, and catfish.

See Box 6-10 for an example of how mercury was used in the hat industry.

BOX 6.10

MAD AS A HATTER

Salt of mercury was once used to flatten felt on hats. Workers in this industry had a higher incidence of a cluster of symptoms: tremors, drooling, and paranoia. This is where the phrase "mad as a hatter" originated.

Mercury is also found in thermometers, medications, lab chemicals, and dental amalgam. Increased concern about mercury's effect on the body revolves around mercury released from dental amalgam during placement. This appears to be a worldwide concern, as research continues to discover a relationship between mercury absorption and disease processes. The American Dental Association's position remains that dental amalgam is safe because mercury binds with silver, copper, and tin into a hard, stable substance.

Counseling Patients

Consider the following when counseling patients:

- Use the same caution in purchasing minerals as with vitamins (see Counseling Patients section in Chapter 5, Vitamins).
- Excessive use of processed food may lead to:
  - deficiencies of calcium, iron, and zinc
  - excess of sodium and chloride
- When preparing food:
  - Although minerals are not destroyed by heat, boiling and stewing cause leaching into surrounding fluid. Use this fluid to prepare rice, mashed potatoes, pasta, etc.
  - Steaming and stir frying retain minerals.
  - Be frugal when adding salt to a prepared meal.
  - Cast-iron cookware adds absorbable iron, especially when cooking acidic foods like tomatoes.

PUTTING THIS INTO PRACTICE

1. Place the labels from the box, package, can, or bottle of your favorite processed foods in front of you. Read the list of ingredients and locate as many minerals as you can. Write down all the minerals that are more than half the daily recommended allowance.
2. Check the label of your daily multivitamin/mineral supplement to determine which minerals and their percentage of RDI it contains. Add the percentage of the minerals in the supplement with the percentage contained in your favorite processed foods to determine your daily consumption.
3. Which minerals are you consuming in excess?
4. Which minerals are deficient in your diet?

CHAPTER QUIZ

1. Potentially toxic minerals are less absorbable than those with a low potential for toxicity.
   a. True
   b. False

2. Phylates and oxylates bind with minerals to enhance their absorption.
   a. True
   b. False

3. Processed foods are high in which of the following minerals?
   a. Calcium and phosphorus
   b. Sodium and chloride
   c. Sulphur and selenium
   d. Potassium and iron

4. Which of the following minerals is essential for glucose metabolism?
   a. Calcium
   b. Chromium
   c. Magnesium
   d. Iodine

5. During an oral examination, you noticed your client had a goiter of the thyroid gland. Goiters form as a result of which mineral deficiency?
   a. Iron
   b. Selenium
   c. Sodium
   d. Iodine

6. Bones and teeth contain what percent of the body's calcium?
   a. 99%
   b. 55%
   c. 25%
   d. 10%

7. Vitamin C helps with the absorption of which mineral?
   a. Calcium
   b. Iron
   c. Sodium
   d. Copper

8. Minerals, like vitamins, can be destroyed during cooking.
   a. True
   b. False

9. Which of the following minerals are considered electrolytes and regulate our fluid balance?

   a. Sodium, potassium, and chloride

   b. Calcium, sodium, and chloride

   c. Sulphur, selenium, and iron

   d. Iron, copper, and zinc

10. Which mineral excess can cause stains of the teeth and deficiency can increase dental caries?

    a. Calcium

    b. Phosphorus

    c. Potassium

    d. Fluoride

Web Resources

Center for Disease Control—Childhood Lead Poisoning Prevention Program http://www.cdc.gov/nceh/lead/lead.htm

Food and Drug Administration, Department of Health and Human Services—Health Care Claims: Sodium and Hypertension http://vm.cfsan.fda.gov/~lrd/cf101-74.html

GlaxoSmithKline Calcium Information http://www.calciuminfo.com

HealthWorld Online, American Institute of Preventive Medicine—Women's Health: Anemia http://www.healthy.net/scr/article.asp?PageType=article&ID=1211

Information From the Heart Foundation—Salt and Hypertension http://www.heartfoundation.com.au/downloads/salt_and_hypertension.pdf

The Linus Pauling Institute—Micronutrient Information Center: Calcium http://lpi.oregonstate.edu/infocenter/minerals/calcium/

Mercury Poisoning News http://www.mercurypoisoningnews.com/

National Dairy Council—Nutrition and Product Information http://www.nationaldairycouncil.org/nutrition/index.asp

National Institute of Health—Facts About Zinc http://www.cc.nih.gov/ccc/supplements/zinc.html

National Osteoporosis Foundation—Calcium and Vitamin D http://www.nof.org/prevention/calcium.htm

National Safety Council—Fact Sheet Library: Lead Poisoning http://www.nsc.org/library/facts/lead.htm

Salt Institute—Citizen Petition: Reaction to the FDA's Paper on Sodium and Hypertension http://www.saltinstitute.org/pubstat/petition.html

Salt Institute—Salt and Hypertension http://www.saltinstitute.org/52.html

U.S. Environmental Protection Agency—FAQ: Lead Poisoning http://www.epa.gov/region02/faq/lead_p.htm

U.S. Environmental Protection Agency—Fish Advisories http://www.epa.gov/ost/fish

U.S. Department of Health and Human Services and U.S. Environmental Protection Agency—What You Need to Know About Mercury in Fish and Shellfish http://www.cfsan.fda.gov/~dms/admehg3.html

The Vegetarian Resource Group—Calcium in the Vegan Diet http://www.vrg.org/nutrition/calcium.htm

References

1. Brody J. A dietary mineral you need and probably didn't know it. New York Times, May 18, 2004.

2. Massé PG, Dosy J, Tranchant CC, Dallaire R. Dietary macro- and micronutrient intakes of nonsupplemented pre- and postmenopausal women with a perspective on menopause associated diseases. J Hum Nutr Diet. 2004;17(2):121–132.

3. Valimaki MJ, Laitinen KA, Tahtela RK, Hirvonen EJ, Risteli JP. The effects of transdermal estrogen therapy on bone mass and turnover in early postmenopausal smokers: a prospective, controlled study. Am J Obstet Gynecol. 2003;189(5):1213–1220.

4. Moyad MA. Calcium oxalate kidney stones: another reason to encourage moderate calcium intakes and other dietary changes. Urol Nurs. 2003;23(4):310–313.

5. Presne C, et al. Randomized trials in the prevention of recurrent calcium stones. Nephrology 2003;24(6):303–307.

6. Curham GC. Dietary factors and the risk of incident kidney stones in younger women: nurses' health study II. Arch Intern Med. 2004;164(8):885–891.

7. Billings RJ, Berkowitz RJ, Watson G. Teeth. Pediatrics 2004;113(4 Suppl):1120–1127.

8. Aoba T, Fejerskov O. Dental fluorosis: chemistry and biology. Crit Rev Oral Biol Med. 2002;12(2):155–170.

9. Fomon SJ, Ekstrand J, Ziegler EE. Fluoride intake and prevalence of dental fluorosis: trends in fluoride intake with special attention to infants. J Public Health Dent. 2000;60(3):131–139.

10. Den Besten PK. Mechanism and timing of fluoride effects on developing enamel. J Public Health Dent. 1999;59(4):247–251.

11. Limdi JK, Crampton JR. Hereditary hemochromatosis. QJM 2004;97(6):315–324.

Suggested Readings

Centers for Disease Control and Prevention. Blood lead levels in residents of homes with elevated lead in tap water—District of Columbia, 2004. MMWR Morb Mortal Wkly Rep. 2004;53(12):268–270.

Davis JR, Stegeman CA. The Dental Hygienist's Guide to Nutritional Care. Philadelphia: W. B. Saunders, 1998.

Diaz JH. Is fish consumption safe? J La State Med Soc. 2004;156(1):42, 44–49.

DuPuy N, Mermel VL. Focus on Nutrition. St. Louis, MO: Mosby, 1995.

Ehrlich A. Nutrition and Dental Health. 2nd Ed. Albany, NY: Delmar, 1995.

Gidlow DA. Lead toxicity. Occup Med. 2004;54(2):76–81.

Katch FI, Katch VL, McArdle WD. Introduction to Nutrition, Exercise, and Health. 4th Ed. Baltimore, Lippincott Williams and Wilkins, 1993.

Logothetis DD. High Yield Facts of Dental Hygiene. Upper Saddle River, NJ: Prentice Hall, 2003.

Morris WC, Knight EL. Nutrition for Dental Hygienists. Lakeland, FL: ISC Wellness Series, 1993.

Needleman H. Lead poisoning. Annu Rev Med. 2004;55:209–222.

Palmer CA. Diet and Nutrition in Oral Health. Upper Saddle River, NJ: Prentice Hall, 2003.

Suzuki Y, Davison KS, Chilibeck PD. Total calcium intake is associated with cortical bone mineral density in a cohort of postmenopausal women not taking estrogen. J Nutr Health Aging 2003;7(5):296–299.

Troost, FJ, Brummer RJM, Dainty JR, Hoogewerff JA, Bull VJ, Saris WHM. Iron supplements inhibit zinc but not copper absorption in vivo in ileostomy subjects. Am J Clin Nutr. 2003;78(5):1018.

Yip HK, Li DK, Yau DC. Dental amalgam and human health. Int Dent J. 2003;53(6):464–468.

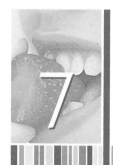

WATER

Vital for Life

Introduction

Water is essential for life, and our need for it is second only to oxygen. Our bodies are 55% to 70% water, and our brains are about 90% water. That amounts to between 10 and 12 gallons. To emphasize its importance: We can survive about 28 days without food but will be in serious trouble after 3 days without water. You would think that if our bodies are mostly water, we would slosh when we walked, but the water is within every body cell, neatly encased by cell walls and membranes. Generally speaking, there is a little bit of water everywhere in our body, but not a lot in any one place.

Absorption and Storage in the Body

Water is freely absorbed, secreted, and reabsorbed in both the small and large intestines. Maintaining homeostasis is very important, because 99% of all our body's chemical reactions depend on water. Fluid within the cells accounts for two-thirds of our body's water, and the rest is outside and between cells as blood plasma and lymph. Figure 7-1 illustrates the flow of water between the two compartments, and Figure 7-2 details the contents of intracellular and extracellular water.

Water is stored intracellularly (65% of body water), where metabolic work takes place, and extracellularly, serving as a transport for nutrients and wastes throughout the body. Water is constantly moving in and out through cell membranes, and the electrically charged minerals of sodium, potassium, and chloride make this possible. This is sometimes referred to as a "pumping action" that maintains homeostasis—water balance—within and between our cells.

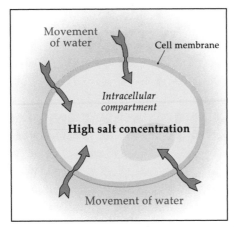 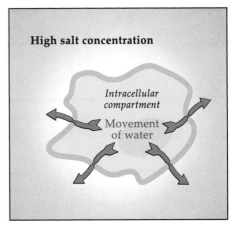

Figure 7-1. Flow of water.

Purpose/Function of Water in the Human Body

- Removes and dilutes toxic waste
- Acts as a solvent to make chemical reactions possible
- Is a major transport system
- Builds tissue
- Regulates body temperature
- Cushions delicate tissues
- Moistens mucous membranes

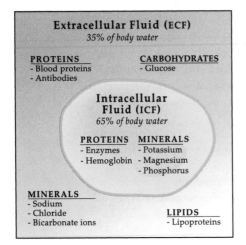

Figure 7-2. Contents of intracellular and extracellular compartments.

Water Acts as a Solvent and Removes Toxic Waste

One of the main functions of water is to provide the solution for metabolic processes to take place and then to remove any toxins produced. Our bodies must remove the waste even in the absence of fluid intake to keep from being poisoned. Total body water loss comes from two-thirds urine and one-third evaporation through the lungs and skin. Kidneys help accomplish this by producing a minimum of one pint of urine each day. We lose approximately two and a half cups of fluid from normal perspiration and up to three gallons or more if exercising for an extended period in a hot climate. Water will also dissolve flavoring compounds and can dilute noxious substances that were accidentally ingested.

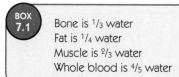

Water Builds Tissue and Acts as a Transport System

Water not only removes toxic and metabolic waste but also delivers nutrients by way of blood and lymph systems. Our blood is four-fifths water. Box 7-1 lists water content of body tissues.

Muscle holds more water than fat. Men generally have leaner muscle mass than women, so generally speaking, the female body has lower water content than the male body. Less muscle mass and higher body fat ratios equal less water. Obese people have smaller percentages of water because body fat does not hold water.

Water Regulates Body Temperature

Water transports heat from one part of the body to another and evaporates from the skin and lungs to control body temperature. Because the body uses water as a coolant, any condition that increases body temperature, such as physical activity or fever, increases the need for water.

Water Cushions and Moistens Delicate Tissues

Water cushions delicate tissues in body structures. Synovial fluid in joints, vitreous fluid in eyes, and fluid in the spinal cord cushions and protects. Water acts as a lubricant to permit movement without friction for our gastrointestinal and respiratory tracts.

Nutrient Intake Standards

Every day, we lose an average of 10 cups of water through normal perspiration, breathing, urination, and feces elimination. This amount must be replaced daily or the body will be in a state of dehydration. At the very least, humans need a little over **one quart** of water each day just to replenish unavoidable losses in urine, feces, sweat, and expired air. Eight 8-oz glasses of water per day for the average *inactive* man or woman has been recommended. Figure 7-3 illustrates the amount of recommended daily water intake.

If this amount is more than you usually drink and you suddenly increase your water intake, you will temporarily increase your frequency of urination. Over time, the body will eventually accommodate the increased water intake without any noticeable side effects.

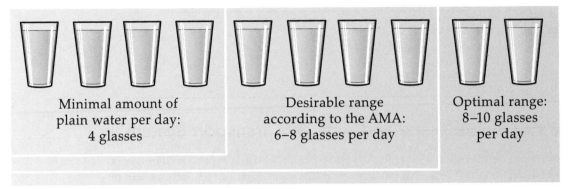

Minimal amount of
plain water per day:
4 glasses

Desirable range
according to the AMA:
6–8 glasses per day

Optimal range:
8–10 glasses
per day

Figure 7-3. Recommended water intake.

Meeting Water Needs

We meet our daily water needs through food and beverages and water created from metabolic processes. Approximately 300 mL of water is released as the body metabolizes carbohydrates, proteins, and lipids; this must also be accounted for when meeting water needs. Drinking water and other beverages supplies the body with most of its required daily intake. Caffeinated beverages such as coffee, tea, and colas can function as a diuretic, causing the body to lose water, but you still end up with some water available from the beverage for bodily functions.

Foods like soup, salads, and fruits and vegetables also supply the body with water. Most foods offer the benefit of some water—even the driest cracker contains almost 3% of water. Fatty foods and those with high sucrose content, however, are not very hydrating, if at all. Boxes 7-2 lists sources of water, and 7-3 offers information regarding solutes in beverages.

BOX 7.2

SOURCES OF DIETARY WATER

$1/3$ comes from foods
$2/3$ comes from beverages

BOX 7.3

ALL BEVERAGES ARE NOT EQUAL

Juice, soft drinks, and soup all add fluid to the body, but they also add solutes that must be diluted as they enter the bloodstream.

Table 7-1 shows approximate water percentages of some common foods.

Water Intoxication

Although water intoxication is uncommon, it can occur. It usually happens when the kidneys are not functioning properly and are unable to excrete water as quickly as needed. Symptoms include headache, nausea, uncoordinated movements with possible progression to unconsciousness, bloating, low body temperature, and seizures. These changes occur because water follows sodium—the excess water dilutes sodium in the blood, causing swelling of cells. This changes the osmotic pressure in tissues as water flows from extracellular fluid into cells. The increase in body fluid can put pressure on the brain, which can lead to seizures or death. This increase also causes the blood volume to drop, which could lead to circulatory shock.

Water Deficiency

Thirst is the first sign of dehydration. Everyone experiences mild dehydration on a daily basis—the headachy, vague feeling that something isn't right. You might feel heartburn, stomach cramps, low-back pain, or fatigue. If not alleviated, thirst can progress rapidly to weakness, exhaustion, delirium, and in the most extreme case, death. Even if water

Table 7-1.   Water Percentages of Common Foods

Food	% Water
Lettuce	98
Celery	96
Watermelon	92
Carrots	90
Milk	88
Oranges	87
Pears	85
Broccoli	85
Apples	84
Peaches	83
Blueberries	80
Beans	79
Eggs	75
Bread	37
Margarine	15
Nuts	5
Crackers	3

balance is restored after significant dehydration, kidneys may have been permanently damaged.

Aging affects our body's need and use of water. Around the age of 35, all five senses and most organ function begin to diminish. We lose the capability to feel thirsty and our body does not conserve water as efficiently.[1] As a result, the elderly are at risk for dehydration. Infants and children are also at risk of dehydration because their bodies contain more water per pound than the bodies of adults.

Dehydrating factors to consider:

- Symptoms include, thirst, dark-yellow urine, difficulty concentrating, and slight headache.
- Caffeinated beverages affect your hormones that regulate the body's fluid balance, causing more urine production.
- Sugar and salt in fruit juices, soups, and soft drinks increase the concentration of solutes in blood. The body's first response is to pull fluid from the cells into the bloodstream to dilute the sugar and salt.
- Nicotine is dehydrating.
- You can lose up to 2 lbs after 3 hours on a plane due to dehydration.

Edema/Water Retention

Edema occurs when water from blood plasma flows out of the circulatory system and into the extracellular spaces between the cells. Sometimes the leakage is severe enough to cause the appearance of a fat belly on a starving child. (Lack of protein promotes water retention in the bloodstream.) An example of mild edema would be when you rise in the morning and your fingers feel swollen or blanch at the knuckles when you try to bend them; this is water retention in the joints and is your body's way of conserving water when it is poorly hydrated. Staying well-hydrated can easily reverse mild instances of edema.

ADH and Water Excretion

An antidiuretic hormone (ADH), secreted from the pituitary gland, affects fluid balance by regulating retention and excretion of water through the kidneys. If minerals become too concentrated in any one compartment of the body, they will pull fluid from other compartments to dilute themselves. Here is an example of how it works:

- You eat pizza and find yourself feeling thirsty.
- Sodium from highly salted food accumulates in the extracellular fluid and pulls water from your cells.
- Sensors in the cells signal your brain of the danger in cellular dehydration and you become thirsty.

- You drink until you no longer feel thirsty.
- By drinking more than the cells need, your body will signal the kidneys to make more urine by filtering the excess fluid out of the blood.

Salt's ability to attract water is the reason it has been used to cleanse wounds and preserve meats. It kills bacteria by dehydrating them.

Potable Water

Potable water is that which is fit to drink. The purest, healthiest, and tastiest water may come out of your tap. New water is not created—it is recycled through a continuous process of precipitation, percolation, and evaporation. Water can be categorized as soft or hard, depending on where it comes from underground and its mineral content. Rainwater and irrigation leach pesticides, herbicides, and fertilizers into the water supply, so it is important to have your drinking water tested periodically.

Soft Water:

- Has a low mineral content
- Comes from sources deep in the ground
- Produces good soapsuds

Hard Water:

- Comes from shallow sources and is usually high in calcium and magnesium
- Reduces the sudsing action
- Produces mineral deposits in pipes, tubs, and sinks, and on clothes and dishware

Table 7-2 compares soft and hard water.

Table 7-2. Soft and Hard Water	
Soft Water	**Hard Water**
Low mineral content	High mineral content
Source deep in the ground	Shallow sources
Good sudsing action	Poor sudsing action
Pipes remain clean	Produces mineral deposits in pipes, tubs, and sinks and on clothes and dishware

Storing Water

If you have to store water for future use, it is best to store it in a container that has been sterilized with Clorox or soaked in a baking soda solution. Glass containers are superior because plastic containers may leach harmful chemicals into the water if exposed to extreme temperatures. Replenish holding containers with new water every few weeks so that bacteria don't grow.

Bottled Water

The U.S. International Bottled Water Association reported yearly profits in excess of 6.4 billion dollars. There are more people buying bottled water than ever imagined 20 years ago, and each year the figures increase. Soda bottlers have ensured their part of the profits by selling water next to their sodas on store shelves. Pepsi bottles Aquafina and Coke bottles Dasani. Over 700 brands of water are offered worldwide. Most bottled water is simply municipal tap water that has been processed for purification and taste.

Environmentalists encourage us to think of the 1.5 million tons of plastic used each year to bottle water. The manufacturing and disposal of plastic bottles releases toxic chemicals into the environment that can create climactic change. Box 7-4 lists common types of drinking water.

Public Water Systems

The Food and Drug Administration (FDA) regulates bottled water, whereas the Environmental Protection Agency (EPA) regulates tap water. The EPA sets safety standards for tap water in the United States, imposing limits on 80 potential contaminants. And though your municipal water supply may meet these limits, it can still make you sick. In 2002, the EPA tested 8,100 of the 55,000 municipal water systems and found that 10% had unsafe levels of lead, which is known to cause permanent neurologic damage. In 2 years the EPA issued over 300,000 violations to water systems around the country for failing to test or treat the water properly. Many municipalities failed to notify the public

---

BOX 7.4 **TYPES OF WATER**

- Tap
- Drinking
- Distilled
- Spring

when known contaminants were at higher-than-safe levels. Even if the contaminants in your tap water meet the minimum requirements, "a lot can happen to your water on the way to the tap,"[2] such as:

- It can become laced with pesticides that are washed into rivers and streams.
- It can be affected by chlorine used to disinfect the water reacting with decaying leaves and forming toxic byproducts.
- It can be contaminated by lead from pipes.

How Safe Is Your Drinking Water?

To learn more about your municipal water supply, contact the EPA hotline at 1-800-426-4791 or visit www.epa.gov/safewater/. You can also investigate by inquiring at your public water utility. The following is a list of the five most widespread contaminants:

- Disinfection byproducts
- Turbidity
- Lead
- Arsenic
- Parasites

You can make your own bottled water by drawing up a container of tap water, boiling it for 10 minutes, and leaving it uncovered and exposed to the air for 24 hours. Chlorine added to the water supply by the municipality (to disinfect) will dissipate into the air. Or, if you so choose, a filter can be installed for safer drinking water. See Table 7-3 for information on water filters.

Distilled Water

Distilled water is processed to remove all minerals and impurities. It is advisable to keep bottles of distilled water capped when not in use because exposure to air causes impurities to be absorbed by the water. Distilled water is not recommended for drinking; there is speculation that when you drink distilled water, it can attract minerals from your body, depleting them as they are excreted in urine.

Spring Water

Spring water comes from a natural spring and contains minerals indigenous to the area. Trace minerals—calcium, magnesium, potassium, phosphorus, copper, and zinc—are sometimes too small to measure. If you want to bottle your own water from a nearby spring, ozonate or disinfect the water before drinking to minimize the possibility of ingesting dangerous bacterium such as *Giardia*.

Table 7-3. Water Filters

Purification System	What It Filters	What It Cannot Filter	Comments
Carbon filter	Pesticides Chlorine	Inorganic chemicals Lead Biologic contaminants	
Ceramic filter	Rust Dirt Parasites	Organic pollutants Pesticides	
Ozone	Bacteria Viruses Algae Parasites	Heavy metals Minerals Pesticides	
UV light	Bacteria Viruses	Heavy metals Pesticides Contaminants	
Ion exchange		Everything	Softens water
Copper-Zinc (KDF)	Copper Zinc	Pesticides Organic contaminants	Chemical reaction releases ozone that kills bacteria, chlorine, and heavy metals; works like a magnet
Reverse Osmosis	90%–98% heavy metals Bacteria Viruses Organic and inorganic chemicals		Wastes 3–8 gallons for every gallon purified
Distillation	Bacteria Viruses Parasites Pathogens Pesticides Herbicides Organic and inorganic chemicals Heavy metals Radioactive contaminants		Uses more electricity than other systems Produces heat when operating Organic chemicals boil at a lower temp than water and will rise to mix with water vapor—ends up in drinking water

Counseling Patients

The American Dental Association recommends that you always inquire about primary and secondary sources of water on health history forms to identify the amount of fluoride ingested in water. It supports the labeling of bottled water with the fluoride concentration of the product and means of contact.

When determining how much water a patient should consume on a daily basis, consider the following:

- The American Dental Association recommends informing patients that:
  - home water treatment systems may remove the fluoride in water
  - bottled water may or may not contain fluoride
- Beverages such as coffee, tea, soda, and alcohol are considered diuretics and actually deplete water stores. If consuming daily, increase water intake accordingly.
- Fruits and vegetables are the food groups that contain high amounts of water.
- Nuts, meats, grains, and fats have some water content, but much lower than that found in fruits and vegetables.
- Assess for xerostomia and salivary flow by having patients chew sugarless gum.
- Teach label reading for hidden sources of sodium.
- Body weight: The more the patient weighs, the more water is needed. Patients should be drinking half their body weight in ounces.
- Age: The very young and old are at greater risk for dehydration. We lose sense of thirst as we age, and preadolescents sweat less than teens and adults, so body temperature rises rapidly during exercise.
- Level of activity and exercise: Patients should sip water every 15 minutes while exercising.
- Weather and climate: Hot climates and fever increase the body's need for water.
- Illness: Fever, diarrhea, and vomiting cause dehydration.
- Pregnancy: Water is needed to support increased blood supply.

Tips for increasing daily water intake:
- Drink an 8-oz glass of water with each meal.
- Take a 16-oz bottle of water when leaving for work and drink it in the car, train, or subway.
- Take a drink of water every time you pass a drinking fountain.
- Drink water while you prepare the evening meal.
- Take a water bottle with you when you exercise.
- Gradually increase the amount you drink to allow your bladder to adjust.
- Fill an empty milk container daily with water and use it to replenish your cup or bottle to keep track of how much you drink.

PUTTING THIS INTO PRACTICE

Tear out this page and take it with you to your local grocery store. Compare the bottled water available to consumers.

1. What types of bottled water are available?

2. If drinking water is available, is it bottled from another municipality in your state?

3. Call your city or county water utility and ask to speak with a chemist. Find out if your water is soft or hard. Ask which minerals are in the water and in what proportion.

4. Write a synopsis of the water purification system and the date of the last treatment center inspection.

5. Write an explanation of the benefits of keeping your body hydrated throughout the day.

6. List some situations that could dehydrate the body.

7. List some benefits to the oral cavity of staying hydrated.

CHAPTER QUIZ

1. Which of the following would be a good source of water as a nutrient?
   a. Food
   b. Coffee and tea
   c. Soda
   d. Alcohol
   e. All of the above

2. If your tap water is soft, there are a lot of natural minerals in the water.
   a. True
   b. False

3. At the very least, how much water does the human body need to replace unavoidable losses?
   a. One gallon
   b. One quart
   c. Ten 8-oz glasses
   d. Half gallon

4. Which type of water is processed to remove all the minerals and impurities?
   a. Tap
   b. Drinking
   c. Distilled
   d. Spring

5. Where is water absorbed in the body?
   a. Small intestine
   b. Large intestine
   c. Kidney
   d. Small and large intestines
   e. Skin pores

6. Aging diminishes the sense of thirst.
   a. True
   b. False

7. The body stores water in which two major compartments?
   a. Intracellular
   b. Extracellular
   c. Intercellular
   d. a and b
   e. b and c

8. The human body requires water to:

   a. Heat itself in cold weather

   b. Transport nutrients and waste

   c. Metabolize carbohydrates and lipids

   d. Maintain a healthy immune system

9. What type of nutrient is water?

   a. Essential

   b. Essential inorganic

   c. Essential organic

   d. Nonessential

10. Edema is an indication of ingestion of too much water.

   a. True

   b. False

Web Resources

International Bottled Water Association www.bottledwater.org

The Public Health and Safety Company (certifies products and writes standards to protect food and water) www.nsf.org

U.S. Environmental Protection Agency www.epa.gov

References

1. DuPuy N, Mermel VL. Focus on Nutrition. St. Louis: Mosby, 1995.

2. Schardt D. Water, water, everywhere. Nutr Action Health Lett. 2000;27(5).

Suggested Readings

Brody J. Must I have another glass of water? Maybe not, a new report says. New York Times, February 17, 2004.

Davis JR, Stegeman CA. The Dental Hygienist's Guide to Nutritional Care. Philadelphia: W. B. Saunders, 1998.

Ehrlich A. Nutrition and Dental Health. 2nd Ed. Albany, NY: Delmar, 1995.

Katch F, McArdle W. Introduction to Nutrition, Exercise, and Health. 4th Ed. Baltimore: Lippincott Williams and Wilkins, 1993.

Logothetis DD. High Yield Facts of Dental Hygiene. Upper Saddle River, NJ: Prentice Hall, 2003.

Policy on Bottled Water, Home Water Treatment Systems and Fluoride Exposure. Adopted by the American Dental Association 2002 House of Delegates.

Why we need water. Available at: www.health24.co.za. Accessed October 2003.

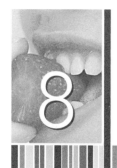

DIETARY AND HERBAL SUPPLEMENTS

8

Uncovering the Unknown

Introduction

In 1994 Congress passed the Dietary Supplement Health and Education Act (DSHEA), which defined and set standards for dietary supplements. These were recognized as products that supplement the diet (not replace food as a sole item of the meal). As such, dietary supplements can be vitamins, amino acids, minerals, herbs, or botanicals and can be in tablet, capsule, powder, tea, softgel, gelcap, or liquid form. This act gave authority to the federal government, more specifically the Food and Drug Administration (FDA), to ensure the safety of supplements and the accuracy of marketing claims. Box 8-1 is a synopsis of the 1994 DSHEA law.

Nutritional supplements sold by the multibillion-dollar nutritional supplement industry are regulated by the FDA and considered food supplements—not drugs. Because of this, advertising restrictions are lax and can mislead the unsuspecting consumer to believe anything the supplement purveyors claim. Separating fact from fiction requires careful research and critical thinking, because marketers have the ability to persuade the public that supplements can cure all kinds of ills and make other potentially false claims. Fortunately, with the passing of the DSHEA, the federal government was

---

BOX 8.1   **1994 DIETARY SUPPLEMENT HEALTH AND EDUCATION ACT**

- Product intended to supplement the diet
- Tablet, capsule, powder, softgel, gelcap, or liquid form
- Not to be used as conventional food or as the sole item of a meal
- Labeled as a dietary supplement

given the authority to ensure our dietary supplements are safe and properly labeled. The FDA is able to stop the sale of any dietary supplement that is:

- adulterated or misbranded
- marketed with false or unsubstantiated claims that it cures or treats disease
- posing a significant or unreasonable risk of injury
- produced in an unclean environment
- unregulated for potency and stability

The following is an example of how false claims can be believed by unsuspecting consumers and how the federal government can exercise its power to protect the public from false and misleading claims:

> Companies started marketing "Vitamin O" with statements substantiating its function. They claimed that oxygen was vital for life, being the single-most necessary substance for living, and that it fit the definition of a vitamin, which is "a substance found in foods and necessary for life, but not usually manufactured by the body." On May 1, 2000, the Federal Trade Commission charged that the companies made false and unsubstantiated health claims in their advertising for this purported nutritional supplement. The defendants' ads claimed that Vitamin O could treat or prevent serious diseases such as cancer and heart and lung disease by enriching the bloodstream with supplemental oxygen. (Release of the Federal Trade Commission: Marketers of Vitamin "O" Settle FTC Charges of Making False Health Claims; Will Pay $375,000 for Consumer Redress.)

Vitamin and Mineral Supplements

In 1999, the Center for Science in the Public Interest (CSPI) reported in their Nutrition Action Newsletter that even if you eat a balanced diet based on the Food Pyramid guidelines, you may not be getting an adequate supply of vitamins and minerals; therefore, it recommended a daily vitamin and mineral supplement. It suggested to choose a supplement that contains no more than 100% of the recommended daily allowance (RDA). Table 8-1 lists nutrients and suggested daily values (DV). Table 8-2 explains specialty vitamins.

According to the Mayo Clinic's information on vitamins and supplements, cost is no indicator of the benefit of the supplement and naturally produced vitamins are not nutritionally superior to synthetic vitamins. The body does not recognize the difference between natural and manmade: Both are utilized with the same efficiency and stored and excreted as the body's needs direct. Box 8-2 contains a kitchen experiment that will help you discover if your body is benefiting from your supplement.

Table 8-1. Daily Values of Nutrients

Nutrient	DV	Amount to look for *
B-1 Thiamin	1.2 mg	100%
B-2 Riboflavin	1.3 mg	100%
B-3 Niacin	16 mg	100% More may cause liver damage.
B-6	1.7 mg	100% More may cause reversible nerve damage.
B-12	2.4 mcg	100% People over 50 yrs lack stomach acid needed to extract B-12 from food—deficiency may cause irreversible nerve damage that can resemble Alzheimer's.
C	90 mg	250–500 mg will saturate the body's tissues. Over 1,000 mg may cause diarrhea.
Folic acid	400 mcg	100% Possibly reduces risk for heart disease and colon cancer Reduces the risk of birth defects
A	3,000 IU	3,000 IU retinol More may increase hip fractures, liver abnormalities, and birth defects. If the label states that vitamin A is from beta-carotene, high doses over 15,000 IU may increase risk of lung cancer in smokers.
D	400 IU	200 IU under 50 yrs 400 IU over 50 yrs because this age group gets too little vitamin D from sunshine 600 IU over 70
E	33 IU	Studies did not show a relationship between larger doses and protection against heart disease and stroke. 800 IU and higher may increase risk of dying.
K	120 mcg	150–250 ideal to reduce hip fractures Interferes with anticoagulant drug therapy
Calcium	1,200 mg	1,000 mg under 50 yrs 1,200 mg over 50 yrs 2,000 mg may increase risk of prostate cancer A day's worth doesn't fit in the pill so take a supplement if not eating calcium-rich foods.
Iron	18 mg	Men and postmenopausal women need less: 0–8 mcg
Magnesium	420 mg	Americans get too little from foods. Deficiency increases risk for diabetes. Over 350 mg from a supplement may cause diarrhea.
Selenium	55 mcg	More than 800 mcg can cause nails and hair to be brittle. 400 mcg is highest safe level.
Zinc and Copper	11 mg .9 mg	40 mg or higher causes body to lose copper. Higher levels of both can depress immune system.
Chromium	35 mcg	
Iodine		Ignore

Table 8-1. Daily Values of Nutrients (continued)

Manganese
Boron
Molybdenum
Chloride
Potassium
Biotin
Pantothenic acid
Phosphorus
Nickel
Tin
Silicon
Vanadium

We get more phosphorus than we need from our diets—too much impairs calcium absorption. These are supplied in plenty in our diets and for some, we're not sure why the human body even needs them.

* Comments taken from "Spin the Bottle," Nutrition Action, 2002.

Table 8-2. Specialty Vitamins

Vitamin Formula	Distinction
Men's	No more than 9 mg iron
Women's	Premenopausal women 18 mg iron Postmenopausal no more than 9 mg
High Potency	At least 2/3 of nutrients have 100% DV
Stress	No evidence that the extra B and C vitamins reduce stress or repair the damage
Seniors	Reduced amounts of iron and vitamin K
Energy	The extra B, C, or E vitamins do not give more energy
Antioxidant	Studies do not suggest that vitamins A, C, and E reduce the risk of cancer or heart disease
Lutein	Need at least 14,000 mcg to reduce cataracts
Ginseng	Does not boost energy
Ginkgo	Sharper thinking not substantiated

BOX 8.2

TRY THIS AT HOME

Place your vitamin, mineral, and herbal supplements in a cup with enough vinegar to cover them. The vinegar represents hydrochloric acid in the stomach and should dissolve your supplements within 30 minutes. If after 30 minutes the supplement is not dissolved, it is probably passing through your system unabsorbed and unutilized.

Consider the following when purchasing a vitamin/mineral supplement:

- Purchase from a place that has a high turnover like Wal-Mart, Kmart, etc.
- Store brands are just as good as the more expensive brands.
- Glass amber bottles are best because they do not allow oxygen or light through.
- A supplement will dissolve in vinegar within 30 minutes.
- Check the expiration date to be sure you have a few months until the bottle expires.
- Check for the USP mark—United States Pharmacopeia, a nongovernmental medical research group. The mark means the supplement has been batch tested for accurate dosage. It does not mean the supplement is safe and effective. Box 8-3 explains the USP mark.

BOX 8.3

USP = UNITED STATES PHARMACOPEIA

Tests supplements for a fee

Means that the supplement dissolves and is made available to the body

Does not mean the supplement is safe or has special benefits

The amount of vitamin or mineral recommended is based on research conducted to discover how much nutrient is needed to perform its specific function. Individual needs differ from small amounts to large quantities. A bell-shaped curve was established for need requirements, and the recommended amount was established so that 95% of the population's needs would be met. Figure 8-1 explains the concept of safe intake.

There are four notable references that are at times used interchangeably, but are slightly different in their origination and intended use. Values for each nutrient may vary, depending on which standard is used:

1. RDA (recommended dietary allowances): established by the Food and Nutrition Board of the Institute of Medicine as recommendations—not requirements—designed to meet the needs of healthy people who eat an ample, varied diet. The value is the average amount based on a bell-shaped curve demonstrating the variability of nutrient needs of the population.

2. RDI (reference daily intake): established by the FDA to use in nutritional labeling, based on the highest 1968 RDAs.

3. DV (daily value): same as RDA—the FDA's recommendation on how much of a certain nutrient to aim for on a daily basis.

4. DRI (dietary reference intake): most recent recommendations established by the Food and Nutrition Board of the Institute of Medicine. Replaces RDA and can be used to update RDI.

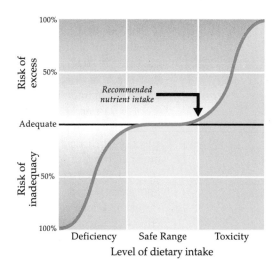

Figure 8-1. Safe intake of nutrients.

Herbal Supplements

Dietary supplements known as herbs consist of plants or parts of plants to flavor, scent, or add therapeutic value to the diet. Because dietary supplements are regulated by the FDA as foods, they do not always meet the same safety and effectiveness standards as prescription and over-the-counter drugs. As a result, some herbal supplements were found to be contaminated with pesticides, metals, microorganisms, and even some prescription drugs. It is wise to buy from a reputable company with a history of supplying superior products.

Most herbal supplements are made from plants, making it difficult to standardize the size of the plant, leaf, or amount of specific active ingredient. It varies quite a bit from one package to the next, and the part of the plant that contains the active ingredient can differ as well, in regard to the seeds, leaves, bark, stem, and flower. The potency of the active ingredient is affected by climate, soil conditions, quality, preparation, and storage.

Reasons for Including Herbal Supplements in the Diet

In a 1998 survey conducted by the American Medical Association, 60 million Americans reported frequent use of herbs. A 2002 survey produced a profile of those most likely to take herbs: educated older women, of average weight, with a healthy lifestyle that included not smoking, exercise, and low-fat diets.[1] The reasons for herbal use are many and varied, so it is important to ensure that herb use is reported on the medical/dental form to better serve our patients. The following are some common reasons for herb usage:

- Failure of traditional medicine to heal
- Lower cost than traditional pharmaceuticals
- Having control over health
- Natural and therefore good for the body

This last statement has sometimes been misconstrued to mean that because herbs are natural they are always safe. This is a false assumption, because many herbs have been proven to cause serious health problems. Adverse reactions to herbs can be serious. One-third of these reactions include heart attacks, liver failure, bleeding, seizures, and death.[2] Of concern to the dental profession is the fact that patients may not be aware that herb consumption should be included on their medical/dental history form. Many herbs interact with traditional medicines, and the health care professional needs to be aware that effects of drugs prescribed could be altered due to herbal medications. Table 8-3 identifies common herbs reported by patients on medical/dental histories.

For various reasons, some patients prefer their dental maladies to be treated with herbs versus traditional medicines and are unaware that some of the herbs can have an effect on their dental treatment. For example, gingko, ginseng, and garlic can prevent blood clotting, causing gingival tissues to bleed freely. Kava kava can enhance anesthesia's sedative effect. St. John's wort should never be taken with other antidepressants. Long-term use of Valerian can increase the amount of anesthesia needed. Ephedra should never be combined with caffeinated beverages because caffeine increases the effects of ephedra. If patients fail to report herb usage, treatment could be compromised, unknowingly to the health care provider. Table 8-4 lists some herbs that are used to treat specific dental conditions.

Table 8-3. Common Herbs Reported on Medical/Dental Histories

Herb	Use	Dental Concern
Aloe	Topical skin lotion	**Interacts with other drugs:** Digoxin Digitalis Thiazide Corticosteroids
Gingko biloba	Improves mental function Improves circulation Tinnitus Vertigo	May cause increased bleeding time **Interacts with other drugs:** Coumadin ASA NSAIDs Plavix Ticlid
Echinacea	Enhances immune system Shortens colds and flu	**Interacts with other drugs:** Cyclosporins Corticosteroids
Ginseng	Increases energy Improves mental function Reduces cholesterol	May cause headaches Increases bleeding time Agitation Insomnia Hypertension Interacts with insulin, NSAIDs, and warfarin
Garlic	Reduces cholesterol Antibiotic Digestive aid Diuretic Expectorant	Thins the blood **Interacts with other drugs:** Warfarin Ticlopidine ASA Heparin
St. John's wort	Relieves depression Relieves uterine cramping Helps fight infection	May cause dry mouth, dizziness, photosensitivity, headache, fatigue **Interacts with other drugs:** Warfarin Prozac, Zoloft, Paxil Tetracycline Cyclosporin Indinavir Digoxin Theophylline
Saw palmetto	Provides relief from enlarged prostate symptoms and irritable bladder	GI upset
Kava kava	Relaxation Diuretic Improves sleeping habits	Visual and hearing impairment Loss of tongue control Exacerbates Parkinson's disease May affect neck muscles so that head becomes twisted
Valerian	Improves sleeping habits	May cause headaches and restlessness May cause increased sedation
Ma-huang (ephedra)	Treats colds and bronchitis Weight loss	Hypertension, tachycardia, heart palpitations, dizziness, insomnia, agitation Increases effects of caffeine

> ## Table 8-4. Herbs Used in Dental Treatment
>
> | Dental Use | Herb |
> |---|---|
> | Soothe inflamed gingival tissues | Aloe, anise, chamomile, eucalyptus, evening primrose, ginseng, golden seal, horsetail, myrrh, peppermint, red clover, rosemary, sage, skull cap, tea tree oil, wintergreen |
> | Relieve halitosis | Anise, clove, parsley, myrrh, rosemary |
> | Relieve pain | Burdock, cayenne, chickweed, cloves, comfrey, marigold, marjoram, peppermint, wintergreen |
> | Relaxation prior to treatment | Catnip, chamomile, hops, red clover, rockrose, sage, skull cap, wood betony |
> | Root canal treatment | Dandelion, echinacea, red clover |
> | Reduce bleeding after extraction | Annatto, Shepard's purse |
> | Relieve pain and pressure after orthodontic adjustment | Comfrey, lobelia, marigold |
> | Antibiotic | Garlic, red clover |
> | Astringent/antiseptic | Wintergreen, witch hazel |
> | Relieve cramps in jaw or neck | Black cohosh, burdock, comfrey |
> | Relief from toothache | Cayenne, hops, marjoram, peppermint |
> | Enhance healing after surgery | Elderberry, tea tree oil, yarrow |
> | Maintenance of healthy oral structures | Kelp |
> | Increases flow of saliva | Prickly ash |
> | Treatment of herpes | Thyme (salve includes other herbs) |
> | Soothes canker sores | Violet |

If a patient reports taking an herb for medicinal treatment or to enhance health, be sure to cross-reference the herb in a table or the PDR Herbal Supplements Index to identify herb-drug interactions. Table 8-5 identifies some of these herb-drug interactions.

Counseling Patients

It is strongly recommended that before taking herbs, you consult with your physician or a professional trained in herb usage. The following suggestions about taking herbal supplements have been taken from Medfacts, a website supported by the National Jewish Medical and Research Center:

1. Research an herbal supplement before taking it.

2. Do not assume a product is safe or effective.

3. Although touted as natural and safe, herbs act as drugs but may lack scientific study.

4. Follow guidelines for dosages and length of time for which the herb can be safely taken.

5. Buy herbs from reliable sources. Labels should include ingredient list, precautions, manufacturer's name and address, batch or lot number, manufacture date, expiration date, and dosage information.

6. Introduce herbs one at a time to monitor effectiveness and side effects. Using multiple herbal supplements puts you at a greater risk for possible adverse reactions.

7. Do not give herbs to infants or young children.

8. Do not take herbs if you are pregnant, nursing, or planning a pregnancy.

9. Use extreme caution with herbs purchased in other countries or through mail order.

10. Herbs can be part of an overall health maintenance program. Before taking, investigate a product thoroughly.[3]

Table 8-5. Herbal/Supplements Interactions

Herbal/Supplements	Interacting Drug, Disease, Foods	Details
Alfalfa	Antacids, H2 antagonists	Mucosal irritation
	Hypoglycemic agents	Hypoglycemic activity
	Anticoagulants	Potentiation, coumarin constituents
	Lipid-lowering drugs	Hypocholesterolaemic in vivo
	Systemic lupus erythematosis	Antagonism, contraindicated
	Hormonal agents	Oestrogenic in vivo
Aniseed	Antihypertensives, MAO inhibitors	Sympathomimetic activity
Borage	Anticonvulsants	Lowered seizure threshold
Caffeine (in cola, ilex, and paullinia preparations)	Pipemidic acid, ciprofloxacin, enoxacin	The antibacterial action of the quinolones inhibits the metabolism of caffeine. Adverse effects of caffeine (tremor, tachycardia) may occur.
Chamomile	Anticoagulants	Potentiation, coumarin constituents
	CNS depressants	Potentiation of sedation
Capsicum	Antacids, H2 antagonists	Mucosal irritation
	Antihypertensives, MAOI inhibitors	Sympathomimetic activity
Celery	Diuretics	Reputed action, potentiation
	Anticoagulants	Potentiation, coumarin constituents
	Cardiac conditions and medications	Hypotensive activity, human and in vivo
	CNS depressants	Potentiation of sedation
	Hypoglycemic agents	Hypoglycemic activity in vivo
Clove	Anticoagulants	Antiplatelet activity, eugenol
Cola, caffeine	Cardiac conditions and medications	Cardioactivity, hypertensive activity
Dandelion	Diuretics	Possible potentiation

Table 8-5. Herbal/Supplements Interactions (continued)

Herbal/Supplements	Interacting Drug, Disease, Foods	Details
Dong quai	Tamoxifen	Antagonism of tamoxifen effects
	Oestrogens	Enhanced oestrogenic effects
	Anticoagulants	Additive risk of bleeding
	Phototoxic drugs	Increased risk of phototoxicity
Echinacea used for >8 weeks	Anabolic steroids	Hepatotoxicity
	Methotrexate	Hepatotoxicity
	Amiodarone	Hepatotoxicity
	Ketoconazole	Hepatotoxicity
Echinacea	Immunosuppressants (corticosteroids, cyclosporin)	Antagonistic effects
	Anabolic steroids, amiodarone, methotrexate, ketoconazole	Additive hepatatoxic effects
	Immunosuppressants	Antagonism of immunosuppressants (theoretical risk)
Eucalyptus	Antacids, H2 antagonists	Mucosal irritation
	Hypoglycemic agents	Hypoglycemic activity in vivo
Evening Primrose	Antipsychotics, antiepileptics	Potential risk of seizure
Fenugreek	Lipid-lowering drugs	Hypocholesterolaemic in vivo
	Anticoagulants	Potentiation, coumarin constituents
	Hypoglycemic agents	Hypoglycemic activity in vivo
	Cardiac conditions and medications	Possible cardioactivity
Feverfew	Anticoagulants	Anticoagulant action
	NSAIDs	Inhibits herbal effect
Garlic	Antacids, H2 antagonists	Mucosal irritation
	Anticoagulants	Potentiation of warfarin
	Lipid-lowering drugs	Hypocholesterolaemic in vivo
	Cardiac conditions and medications	Hypotensive activity
	Hypoglycemic agents	Hypoglycemic activity in vivo
Gentian	Hypertension	Possible potentiation
Ginger	Hypertension	Hypertensive activity
	Hypoglycemic agents	Hypoglycemic activity in vivo
	Lipid-lowering drugs	Hypocholesterolaemic in vivo
	Anticoagulants	Inhibition of platelet activity

Table 8-5. Herbal/Supplements Interactions (continued)

Herbal/Supplements	Interacting Drug, Disease, Foods	Details
Gingko biloba	Anticoagulants	Altered bleeding time
Ginseng	Cardiac conditions and medications such as digoxin	Cardioactivity, hypotensive and hypertensive activity. Interference with pharmacodynamics and drug level monitoring
	Anticoagulants	Reduction of blood coagulation
	Insulin, sulphonylureas, biguanides	Altered glucose concentrations—do not prescribe for people with diabetes
	CNS depressants and stimulants, MAOIs	Potentiation of sedation and stimulation, potentiation of MAO inhibition, suspected phenelzine interaction
	Oestrogens	Additive effects
	Corticosteroids	Additive effects
Golden seal (Yellow root)	Cardiac conditions and medications	Cardioactivity, hypotensive activity. Contraindicated in people with raised blood pressure
	CNS depressants	Potentiation of sedation in vivo
	Heparin	Heparin antagonist
Guar gum	Antibacterials	Reduced absorption of penicillin V
Hawthorn	Digoxin	Interference with pharmacodynamics and drug level monitoring
Horseradish	Thyroid hormone	Altered thyroid hormone activity
Karela	Insulin, sulphonylureas, biguanides	Altered glucose concentrations—do not prescribe for people with diabetes
Kava	Benzodiazepines	Additive CNS depression
	Dopamine antagonists	Increased risk of parkinsonism, extrapyramidal symptoms
Kelp	Thyroxine	Iodine content of herb may interfere with thyroid replacement
Kyushin	Digoxin	Interference with pharmacodynamics and drug level monitoring
Licorice	Hypertension, antihypertensives (spironolactone)	Hypertensive and mineralocorticoid activity (antagonizes diuretic effect)
	Anticoagulants	Inhibition of platelet activity
	Digoxin	Interference with pharmacodynamics and drug level monitoring

Table 8-5. Herbal/Supplements Interactions (continued)

Herbal/Supplements	Interacting Drug, Disease, Foods	Details
	Glucose intolerance	Reduced potassium aggravates glucose tolerance
	Hormonal agents	Oestrogenic in vivo
	Prednisolone	Glycyrrhizin decreases plasma clearance of prednisolone and increases plasma prednisolone concentrations and AUC
	Hydrocortisone	Glycyrrhetinic acid (metabolite of glycyrrhizin) potentiates cutaneous vasoconstrictor response of hydrocortisone
	Oral contraceptives	May increase sensitivity to glycyrrhizin, causing hypertension, edema, and hypokalaemia. Women are reportedly more sensitive than men to the adverse effects of licorice.
Myrrh	Thyroid hormone	Altered thyroid hormone activity
Parsley	Antacids, H2 antagonists	Mucosal irritation
	Cardiac conditions and medications	Hypotensive activity
	MAOIs	Possible potentiation
Plantain	Digoxin	Interference with pharmacodynamics and drug level monitoring
Psyllium (plantago ovata)	Lithium	Decreased lithium concentrations (hydrophilic psyllium may prevent lithium from ionizing)
Red clover	Hormonal agents	Oestrogenic in vivo
	Anticoagulants	Potentiation, coumarin constituents
Saiboku-to (Asian herbal mixture; contains same herbs as sho-saiko-to, xiao chai hu tang, Poria cocos, Magnolia officinalis, Perillae frutescens)	Prednisolone	Increased prednisolone AUC
Saw palmetto	Hormonal agents	Oestrogenic and antiandrogenic in vivo
Senega	Antacids, H2 antagonists	Irritant saponins
Shankhapushpl (Ayurvedic mixed-herbs)	Phenytoin	Decreased phenytoin concentrations, loss of seizure control

Table 8-5. Herbal/Supplements Interactions (continued)

Herbal/Supplements	Interacting Drug, Disease, Foods	Details
Sparteine in Cytisus scoparius	Quinidine, haloperidol, moclobemide	Quinidine is a potent inhibitor of the oxidative metabolism of sparteine. Similar effects have been observed with haloperidol and moclobemide. Substantial doses of sparteine in slow metabolizers may cause adverse effects such as circulatory collapse.
St John's wort	HIV protease inhibitors (indinavir, nelfinavir, ritonavir, saquinavir)	Reduced blood levels with possible loss of HIV suppression
	Immunosuppressants (cyclosporins, tacrolimus)	Reduced blood levels with transplant rejection
	HIV nonnucleoside inhibitors (efavirenz, nevirapine, delavirdine)	Reduced blood levels with possible loss of HIV suppression
	Anticonvulsants (carbamazepine, phenobarbitone, phenytoin)	Reduced blood levels with risk of seizures theoretically possible
	Digoxin	Reduced blood levels with theoretical loss of control of heart rhythm or heart failure
	SSRIs and related antidepressants (citalopram, fluoxetine, fluvoxamine, paroxetine, sertraline, nefazodone)	Increased serotonergic effects
	Triptans (sumatriptan, naratriptan, rizatriptan, zolmitriptan)	Increased serotonergic effects with theoretical chances of adverse reactions
	Oral contraceptives	Breakthrough bleeding. Contraceptive failure theoretically possible
	Theophylline	Reduced blood levels and loss of bronchodilator effect theoretically possible
	Iron	Tannic acid of herbs might limit iron absorption
	Piroxicam, tetracyclines	Increased phototoxicity
	Phenprocoumon	Decreased phenprocoumon AUC
Tamarind (Tamarindus indica)	Aspirin	Increased bioavailability of aspirin
Tumeric	Anticoagulants	Altered bleeding activity
Uva ursi	Diuretics	Reputed action, potentiation
Uzara root	Digoxin	Interference with pharmacodynamics and drug level monitoring

Table 8-5. Herbal/Supplements Interactions (continued)

Herbal/Supplements	Interacting Drug, Disease, Foods	Details
Valerian	CNS depressants	Potentiation of sedation
	Alcohol	A mixture of valepotriates reduces the adverse effects of alcohol on concentration.
Willow bark	Anticoagulants	Salicylate constituents, anticoagulant activity
	Methotrexate, acetazolamide Probenecid	Increased risk of toxicity, salicylate Risk of inhibition of probenecid
Yohimbine (Pausinystalia yohimbine)	Tricyclic antidepressants	Hypertension
Zinc	Immunosuppressants (corticosteroids, cyclosporin)	Antagonistic effects

Reproduced with permission from MediMedia (NZ) Ltd. OTC Medicines Guide, 2003. Available at: www.everybody.co.nz.

PUTTING THIS INTO PRACTICE

Your client is a 28-year-old male with a 3-year history of HIV. His medical/dental history indicates use of prescription drugs and herbs. He is taking the usual protease inhibitors (indinivir) prescribed by his physician and self-medicates with St. John's wort to relieve mild depression. Upon oral exam, you note red and edematous gingival tissues that bleed freely upon probing, slow-acting salivary glands, and light retentive plaque.

1. Explain to your client the interaction of indinivir and St. John's wort.
2. What other oral symptoms are caused by St. John's wort that could have an overall effect on active disease?
3. What recommendations might the dentist make to this client to improve his oral health?

CHAPTER QUIZ

1. Herbal supplements are very safe to the human body because they are made from plants and other compounds naturally found in nature.
   a. True
   b. False

2. The USPS seal on the supplement bottle means:
   a. The contents are safe and effective.
   b. The comments on the label are true about curing certain disease states.
   c. The supplement will dissolve and be made available for use by the body.
   d. The supplement was manufactured and packaged under federal supervision.

3. Herbal supplements containing the USPS seal are safe for children and pregnant women.
   a. True
   b. False

4. Which of the following statements is true when considering vitamin/mineral supplements?
   a. Premenopausal women require more iron than postmenopausal women.
   b. Men require less iron than postmenopausal women.
   c. Children and infants require more iron than any other age group.
   d. Men and women under 50 require less iron than those over 50.

5. Which of the following herbs is sometimes substituted for antibiotics?
   a. Willow bark
   b. Ephedra
   c. Garlic
   d. Marjoram

6. If a client wanted quick relief from toothache pain, which of the following herbal remedies might she try?
   a. Wintergreen
   b. Cayenne
   c. Black cohosh
   d. Aloe

7. Overdosing on selenium may cause hair and nails to become brittle.
   a. True
   b. False

Web Resources

Food and Drug Administration Guide on Herbs
http://vm.cfsan.fda.gov/~dms/fdsupp.html
http://www.nal.usda.gov/fnic/etext/000015.html
http://vm.cfsan.fda.gov/~dms/supplmnt.html

General Information on Herbal Supplements
http://www.nlm.nih.gov/medlineplus/herbalmedicine.html
http://www.nutritional-supplement-info.com/
http://www.nutritional-supplement-guide.com/html/herbal_supplements.html
http://www.herbmed.org/
http://www.mskcc.org/mskcc/html/11570.cfm
http://www.citizen.org/hrg/drugs/articles.cfm?ID=5195
http://healthlink.mcw.edu/article/964721794.html

Information on Herb and Drug Interactions
http://www.everybody.co.nz/otc/herbals.html

Information on Herbs Contraindicated During Pregnancy and Lactation
http://www.marchofdimes.com/professionals/681_1815.asp
http://www.marchofdimes.com/pnhec/159_529.asp

Information on Herbs—National Jewish Hospital
http://www.nationaljewish.org

Information on Herbs—Mayo Clinic
http://www.cnn.com/HEALTH/library/NU/00205.html

Information on Side Effects, Warnings, and Drug Interactions
http://www.consumerlab.com/recalls.asp
http://www.personalhealthzone.com/herbsafety.html
http://www.consumersunion.org/pub/core_product_safety/000285.html
http://www.hon.ch/News/HSN/511204.html
http://www.tufts-health.com/RxIQ/RxIQ.php?sec=vitaherb&content=vitamins
http://nccam.nih.gov/health/supplement-safety/
http://www.hc-sc.gc.ca/english/protection/warnings/2002/2002_46e.htm

References

1. Biron C. Herbs: efficacy, adverse reactions, and drug interactions. RDH 2004;64–66,92.

2. Schardt D. Are your supplements safe? Nutr Action Healthletter November 2003:3–7.

3. National Jewish Medical and Research Center, Medfacts. Using herbal supplements wisely. Available at: www.nationaljewish.org.

Suggested Readings

Abebe W. An overview of herbal supplement utilization with particular emphasis on possible interactions with dental drugs and oral manifestations. Journal Dent Hyg. 2003;77(1): 37–46.

Council for Responsible Nutrition. Historical Comparison of RDIs, RDAs and DRI, 1968 to Present. Washington, D.C., 2001.

Danner V. The natural life. Access. April 2001.

Dietary Supplement Bureau. How dietary supplements are regulated. Available at: www.supplementinfo.org. Accessed October 2003.

Duke J. A guide to herbal alternatives. Herbs for Health November/December 1997.

Genger T. Spin the bottle, Nutrition Action Healthletter January/February, 2003.

Katch F, McArdle W. Introduction to Nutrition, Exercise, and Health. 4th Ed. Baltimore: Lippincott Williams and Wilkins, 1993.

National Center for Complimentary and Alternative Medicine, National Institute of Health. Herbal supplements; consider safety, too. Bethesda, MD, 2003.

Office of Dietary Supplements, National Institute of Health. What are dietary supplements. 2003.

Parsa-Stay F. The complete book of dental remedies. Garden City Park, NY: Avery Publishing Group, 1996.

Sherman R. Herbal supplements: implications for dentistry. Presented at the Hawaiian Dental Forum, Honolulu, 2003.

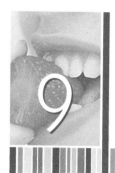

DIET AND DENTAL CARIES

Introduction

The relationship between sugar and dental caries has been well-established: What we include in our diet can have an impact on the health of our teeth. Many of those who aren't in the dentistry field will simply say "sugar gives you cavities," but sugar consumption in the United States has increased while the incidence of dental caries has decreased. If there is a direct cause and effect between the two, then why has there been a decrease in caries? Three reasons: exposure of developing and erupted teeth to fluoride, better oral hygiene practices, and protective factors in saliva. Dental caries is a multifactorial disease dependent on host and diet, but other factors can buffer the effects of sugar on teeth and lessen our chances of developing dental caries.

Humans have long been interested in the taste of sweetness. Evidence of sugar consumption appears as early as 2600 BC in Egyptian tomb drawings depicting beekeepers harvesting honey for the privileged class. By the 1960s, the United States was converting glucose into cornstarch and fructose, which led to the production of high fructose corn syrup, a common ingredient in manufactured foods. This was considered great progress, as fructose is twice as sweet as glucose and half the cost.

Some interesting facts about sugar consumption patterns:

- Sucrose is still the number one choice for tabletop sweetener.
- Males consume more sugar than females.
- The larger the family, the lower the consumption of sugar.
- Teenagers are the greatest consumers, with 15- to 18-year-old males at the top.

Sugar and Caries

It is not completely accurate to state that "sugar" causes cavities. All carbohydrates can demineralize tooth enamel, and sugar—or, rather, sucrose—is only one of many sugars.

Even though a potato chip does not in any way resemble a piece of sweet candy, it can actually be more detrimental to tooth enamel than a teaspoon of sugar. How can this be? A potato chip is a "cooked starch," one form of carbohydrate. Salivary amylase breaks down the starch to a disaccharide that is used by plaque bacteria, resulting in acid production for as long as the potato chip remains in the mouth. Think back to the last time you ate a potato chip, piece of bread, rice, or cracker. Do they not get stuck between your teeth and hang around longer than a piece of hard candy? Then imagine a piece of bread spread with sweet jelly stuck between your teeth. That combination is perhaps the most detrimental of all to your teeth—starch with a sugar. So yes, sugar does cause dental caries, but so do other carbohydrates.

Famous Vipeholm Study

Much of what we know today about the relationship between sugar and dental caries was discovered as a result of a study conducted from 1945 to 1953, involving 436 residents at a mental institution in Vipeholm, Sweden. The study was conducted to see if form and frequency of eating sugar had any effect on dental caries. Residents were divided into different groups receiving varying amounts and forms of sugar, either with their regular meals or between meals as snacks.

- All groups received the basal diet (no simple sugars).
- Another group ate the basal diet with 300 g of additional sugar in solution during meals.
- Another group ate the basal diet with an additional 50 g of sugar in bread with their meals.
- Another group ate the basal diet with in-between-meal snacks of toffee and candy consisting of a small amount of sugar.

The group with the in-between-meal sugared snacks reported the highest caries rate. Based on these 8 years of study, it was determined that:

1. **Frequency** of sugar eaten is the prime factor in caries activity.
2. **Form** and composition of sweets is important: Foods that stayed in the oral cavity and took longer to clear than liquids increased the rate of caries.
3. **Quantity** of sugar eaten is not of great importance: An increase from 30 g to 330 g per day caused little increase in caries production.
4. Sugar exerts caries-promoting effects locally on tooth surfaces.

Factors of Caries Development

Box 9-1 lists six factors that determine the caries susceptibility of a tooth. Variations within the factors can change the incidence and prevalence of dental caries. Bacteria, carbohydrates, and dry mouth all contribute to enamel demineralization. Buffering action of ample saliva, fluoride, and controlling bacteria that help with the caries process all

**BOX
9.1**

SIX FACTORS THAT DETERMINE THE CARIES SUSCEPTIBILITY OF A TOOTH

- Specific bacteria found in dental plaque
- Susceptible tooth structure
- Carbohydrates in the diet
- Saliva
- Absence of fluoride
- Poor oral hygiene

remineralize enamel. Finding a balance between the demineralization and remineralization factors is part of caries risk assessment.

Bacteria Responsible for Formation of Dental Caries

Streptococcus mutans and *Lactobacillus* are just two of over 500 bacteria found living in dental plaque and are the two main bacteria involved in caries formation. The presence of *Streptococcus mutans* is needed to initiate pit and fissure, smooth surface, and root surface decay. *Streptococcus mutans* starts the process and takes it to the enamo-dentin junction, where *Lactobacillus* takes over, extending the lesion into the dentin.

Tooth Structure

Posterior molars with shallow grooves are less susceptible to dental caries because they do not retain plaque and food as do molars with very deep grooves. Teeth with deeper grooves retain plaque and food because toothbrush bristles cannot reach to the depth during daily cleaning. Teeth that are rotated or crowded offer protected areas for plaque to grow and are not cleansed by chewing action or quick toothbrushing. The action of chewing has a cleansing effect on teeth that are all in alignment and with shallow grooves.

**BOX
9.2**

BACTERIA RESPONSIBLE FOR DENTAL CARIES

- *Streptococcus mutans*
- *Lactobacillus*

Host Resistance to Caries:

- Teeth with shallow pits and fissures are less susceptible.
- Straight teeth are less susceptible.
- Caries-resistant tooth anatomy may be influenced by preeruptive nutrition, as certain nutrient deficiencies during fetal development can cause crowded or rotated teeth.
- Newly erupted teeth are more susceptible to decay because enamel is not completely mineralized.

Carbohydrates

All foods and beverages that contain carbohydrates have the potential to cause dental caries. Plaque bacteria feed on carbohydrates and produce acid that can demineralize enamel. Some foods are naturally acidic and erode enamel.[1] If acid byproducts from metabolized carbohydrates or acidic foods drop the normally basic pH of the mouth to below 5.5, enamel demineralization begins. Box 9-3 identifies five different acids that are created when carbohydrates are metabolized by bacteria.

The drop in pH starts within seconds and can become critical in about 5 minutes. The demineralization continues until the pH of the mouth is returned to 7.0 (basic).

Cariogenic Properties of Carbohydrates

Sticky foods such as caramels, jellybeans, gumdrops, and other chewy candies are the foods usually perceived as being most cariogenic. The truth, however, is that cookies, crackers, and potato chips are probably more cariogenic because they are retained longer in the mouth, allowing oral bacteria to metabolize the carbohydrate, producing acid to demineralize enamel. The bacteria feed and make acid for as long as the food remains in the oral cavity. Starch is the least cariogenic of carbohydrates because it is such a large molecule and must be broken down before it can diffuse through plaque, but it is still cariogenic because of its more retentive consistency. Consuming foods containing both starch and sugar may be more cariogenic than those with just simple sugars, because

BOX 9.3

FIVE ACIDS CREATED WHEN CARBOHYDRATES ARE METABOLIZED BY BACTERIA

- Lactic
- Formic
- Proprionic
- Acetic
- Buturic

> ## FACTORS THAT DETERMINE THE CARIOGENICITY OF THE DIET
>
> Physical Form:
>   Liquid
>   Solid
>   Sticky
>
> Frequency of eating events.
>
> Sequence in which foods are eaten.

starch and sugar together hang around longer, giving bacteria a longer time to produce acid from the readily available sugar.

- Monosaccharides and disaccharides are the most cariogenic carbohydrates.
- Sucrose is the most cariogenic of all carbohydrates.
- Starch is the least cariogenic carbohydrate.
- Starch eaten with sucrose (e.g., toast with jelly) is more cariogenic that either one alone because starchy foods stick to the teeth longer.
- Natural sugars such as honey, molasses, and raw sugar (turbinado) are just as cariogenic as refined sugars.
- Corn syrups added to foods are just as cariogenic as refined sugars.
- Honey may be more cariogenic because of its thick and sticky properties.
- Powdered sugar is more cariogenic because it is concentrated and fine.
- Fruits and vegetables and their juices are not as cariogenic as sucrose because of water dilution.
- A food that is 80% sucrose may not be any more harmful than one that is 40% sucrose.

Box 9-4 lists factors that determine the cariogenicity of the diet.

- Physical form: Liquids clear the oral cavity faster than solid or sticky foods.
- Frequency of eating events: Sugary foods eaten 20 minutes apart or on either side of a meal are separate opportunities for bacteria to feed and produce acid.
- Sequence of foods eaten.

Box 9-5 lists protective factors of foods.

- Fats and proteins eaten in the meal may put a coating on the tooth to protect it from sugars eaten later.
- Consuming dairy products keeps the saliva rich in calcium and phosphorus, offering the benefit of remineralization.
- Cheese eaten after a sugar prevents the pH from dropping below 5.5.

BOX 9.5

PROTECTIVE FACTORS OF FOODS

- Fats
- Proteins
- Phosphates
- Fluoride

Fluoride

If a patient reports heavy consumption of sugar, presence of fluoride will reduce its detrimental effect on teeth.[2] Ingestion of fluoride, either in food or water, will increase the fluoride content of saliva, making it available to remineralize enamel. Salivary fluoride levels are elevated for up to 3 hours after brushing with fluoridated toothpaste, bathing teeth, and remineralizing enamel. Fluoride can also accumulate in plaque fluid, offering protective factors adjacent to enamel surfaces.[3,4]

Saliva

After fluoride, saliva is the number one protector of teeth.[3–5] Saliva is saturated with calcium, phosphate, sodium bicarbonate, and proteins. Calcium and phosphate are components of enamel and can repair demineralized areas. Sodium bicarbonate (baking soda) has a high pH and can neutralize acids in the mouth that demineralize enamel. Saliva also "washes" or clears solid and liquid foods from the oral cavity, reducing the amount of time bacteria can feed on carbohydrates and manufacture acid. Saliva dilutes acids and carries them out with the flow of saliva. A multifunction protein in saliva called SLPI has antiviral, bacterial, and fungal properties that reduce and render ineffective the caries causing bacteria in plaque.[5] Eating crunchy or chewy foods will increase salivation and are therefore most desirable. Consuming at least one chewy or crunchy food at each meal is recommended.

Salivary Factors:

- Physical
  - Saliva rinses teeth free of food particles, especially if forced around and in between teeth.
  - Viscous saliva is not as effective as more fluid saliva at rinsing teeth.
  - If a client has an abundance of saliva, food clears the oral cavity faster and so pH will return to 7.0 more quickly.

- Chemical
  - Saliva has sodium bicarbonate, which buffers acid at the plaque/enamel interface.
  - Saliva has calcium and phosphorus, which remineralizes enamel.
  - A protein called sialin in saliva reduces the amount pH drops and also helps the oral pH return to 7.0 quicker.
  - As saliva flow is stimulated (by chewing firm foods) and the amount of saliva increases, there is an increase of remineralizing, buffering, and antibacterial components.
- Antibacterial
  - Mucins in saliva trap bacteria and remove it with normal swallowing patterns.
  - Proteins in saliva are antibacterial.

Oral Hygiene

The motivation and ability to remove bacterial plaque plays a major role in keeping teeth free from dental caries. To increase the number of bacteria in the mouth, plaque must be left on the teeth and carbohydrates must be eaten. When carbohydrates are eaten, plaque becomes stickier and more food is stored to support more bacteria, providing more places for bacteria to exist. Scrupulous home care that removes bacterial plaque on a daily basis eliminates that component in the caries equation.

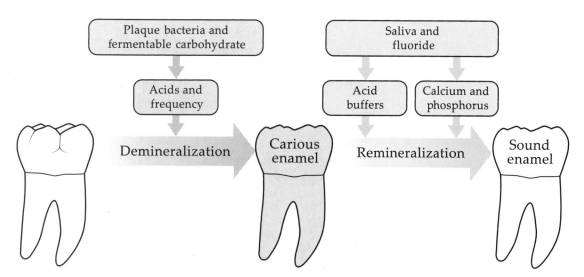

Figure 9-1. Dental caries equation.

Dental Caries Equation

- Plaque holds bacteria close to the enamel.
- When carbohydrates are eaten, they diffuse through the plaque and are metabolized by plaque bacteria.
- The end product is acid.
- Lactic acid production causes the pH at the plaque/enamel interface to drop from 7.0 to less than 5.5 within seconds.

Quick Dental Caries Facts

- If plaque is immature and not very thick, saliva may penetrate plaque and buffer the acid.
- As plaque thickens, saliva cannot buffer acid as easily.
- Acid production continues until carbohydrates are cleared from the mouth.
- Demineralization stops when carbohydrates are cleared.
- Once food is cleared and acid production stops, remineralization can begin.
- If the client uses fluoridated toothpaste or drinks fluoridated water, the remineralized area may be stronger than before.

Early Childhood Caries (ECC)

Figures 9-2 through 9-6 show varying forms of ECC, also known as "bottle-mouth" caries, on children of different ages.

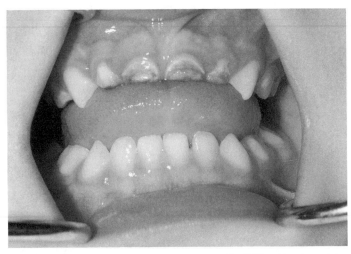

Figure 9-2. Mild form of early childhood caries. (Courtesy of Dr. William Chambers, Asheville, NC.)

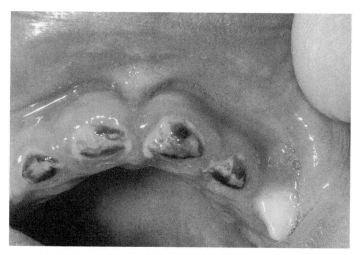

Figure 9-3. Early childhood caries on an 18-month-old child. (Courtesy of Dr. William Chambers, Asheville, NC.)

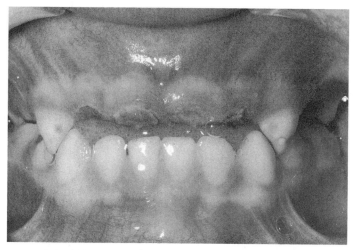

Figure 9-4. Early childhood caries on a 2-year-old child. (Courtesy of Dr. William Chambers, Asheville, NC.)

In 1994, the Center for Disease Control (CDC) changed the name of bottle-mouth caries to early childhood caries, declaring the former name to be too misleading. Early childhood caries can be diagnosed if decay is present on one or more smooth surfaces, but is usually seen as extensive decay of all deciduous teeth, in children 5 years old and younger.[6] Sometimes the mandibular anterior teeth are spared because they are protected by the tongue and saliva. It was believed to occur when a child was put to bed with a bottle of milk or sweetened drink, hence the name "bottle-mouth" caries, but recent studies show that children with ECC have more *Streptococcus mutans* bacteria in their

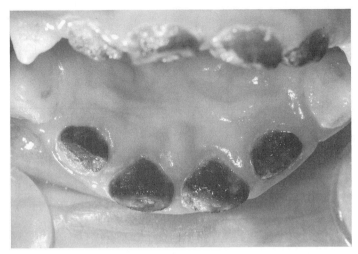

Figure 9-5. Early childhood caries on a 3-year-old child. (Courtesy of Dr. William Chambers, Asheville, NC.)

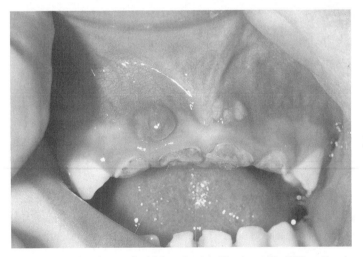

Figure 9-6. Abscesses from early childhood caries. (Courtesy of Dr. William Chambers, Asheville, NC.)

mouths than children without caries. Bacteria feed on the milk (carbohydrate), produce acid, and demineralize enamel. Children quit sucking when they fall asleep, allowing whatever is in the bottle—formula, milk, juice, breast milk—to pool around teeth, thus beginning the demineralization process. Because saliva production slows during sleep, the protective factors of saliva are not available. The American Academy of Pediatric

Dentists recognizes ECC as an epidemic, especially in populations of ethnic minorities. There have been reports that breastfeeding can cause dental caries, but according to studies conducted by the National Institute of Dental and Craniofacial Research, breast-fed children are less likely to develop this disease than those who are fed by bottle. ECC can be prevented if the child is weaned from the bottle by around 9 months old or if they are fed before being put to bed. More importantly, however, daily removal of bacterial plaque by brushing or wiping contributes more to preventing ECC. It is suggested to fill the bottle with plain water if a child must be put to bed with a bottle.

Protective Factors in Food

Cariostatic foods are those that do not contribute to initiation of demineralization or continue the caries process. Some foods and nutrients have cariostatic properties and can actually help prevent dental caries.

- Fats do not lower oral pH to an acidic level and can actually increase the pH after consuming carbohydrates. Fats in the meal should be eaten before sugary dessert.

- Proteins elevate salivary urea, which buffers acid. It has been found that if high-protein foods are eaten after a carbohydrate, the pH returns to 7.0 more quickly. The sequence in which foods are eaten may make a difference—a little bite of cheese, a little bit of sugar, a little bite of cheese, etc. Protein in the meal, like fats, should be eaten before sugary dessert.

- Phosphates also buffer acid. In animal studies where phosphates were added to the diet along with sugar, caries did not occur, but phosphates' cariostatic activity had no lasting effect as fluoride did.

- Fluoride has protective factors that can continue well after the meal has been eaten. Fluoride is naturally occurring in small quantities in some foods such as tea and seafood. The fluoride from the food, water, or beverage makes its way to the saliva, where it bathes the teeth and infiltrates plaque, protecting teeth from acid attacks. Fluoride has both antibacterial and antiplaque capabilities.

Sugar Substitutes

Sugar substitutes are a multimillion-dollar industry. Synthetic sweeteners like saccharine, aspartame, and sugar alcohols are used in many foods to reduce sugar's caries-causing potential.[7] Both synthetic sweeteners and sugar alcohols are noncariogenic, but only the synthetic sweeteners are noncaloric.

Placed next to regular table sugar, sugar alcohols are visually the same, but they are different in that they do not raise blood glucose levels as table sugar does. Sugar alcohols are made by adding hydrogen atoms to sugar. When sugar alcohol enters the intestines, it can cause cramping, bloating, and diarrhea. Because of this, the FDA mandates that manufacturers place a laxative effect warning on labels.

Examples of Sugar Alcohols:

- Xylitol is the alcohol form of xylose and is the most desirable of all sugar substitutes for two reasons:

1. Bacterial plaque does not metabolize xylitol.
2. Xylitol has the ability to reduce salivary *strep mutans* in the mouth.[2]

University of Michigan researchers found that school children who chewed gum with xylitol for 5 minutes, three to five times a day, not only reduced caries but also remineralized incipient lesions.[8] Xylitol occurs naturally in straw, corncobs, fruit, vegetables, cereals, mushrooms, and some seaweed and is made from birch tree chips in Europe and corn stalks in the United States. It has the same sweetness as sucrose.

- Sorbitol is an alcohol form of sucrose made by adding hydrogen to glucose. Research concludes that chewing gum with sorbitol after eating significantly reduced incidence of dental caries.[9]

  Sorbitol occurs naturally in fruits and vegetables and is manufactured from corn syrup.

- Maltitol is the alcohol form of mannose and naturally occurs in pineapples, olives, asparagus, sweet potatoes, and carrots. It is extracted from seaweed for use in manufacturing.

Lesser-known Sugar Alcohols:

- Mannitol
- Lactitol
- Isomalt
- Erythritol

Synthetic Sweeteners

The FDA approves sugar substitutes for use in foods and beverages after extensive animal studies have been conducted to determine if it is safe for human consumption. The most commonly used sweeteners are aspartame, saccharin, and sucralose.

- Aspartame (NutraSweet, Equal, or Nutra Taste) is 180 times sweeter than sucrose and is used by over 100 million people worldwide. Aspartame is made of aspartic acid and the amino acid phenylalanine. It is toxic to those with phenylketonuria (PKU). Many people claim to have adverse reactions—anywhere from forgetfulness or brain fog to seizures and migraines. Research has found these claims to be unfounded. Neotame is made of the same ingredients as aspartame but is more stable and is not metabolized by the body as aspartame is.

- Saccharin (Sweet 'N Low) is 300 times sweeter than sucrose and was at one time considered unsafe. In 1977, the FDA tried to ban saccharin because animal studies showed it caused cancer of the bladder, the reproductive organs, and other vital organs. A warning notice was put on Sweet 'N Low packets and on some food products containing saccharin. In the late 1990s, the Calorie Control Council had Congress reverse the adverse warning when they proved humans and rats do not develop cancer in the same manner. Research on saccharin continues. As recently as 2002, a study proved that consumers who drank more than two diet drinks per day or used more than six packets of saccharin daily had a small increased chance of developing bladder cancer.[10]

- Sucralose (Splenda) is the only sugar substitute made from sugar and is made by chlorinating sucrose. It remains stable at high temperatures, making it an ideal substitute for sugar in recipes. Users report no bitter aftertaste as with saccharin and aspartame. Sucralose is produced by chemically changing the structure of sugar molecules by substituting three chlorine atoms for three hydroxyl groups. With this chemical change, the body is unable to burn sucralose for energy. In 1976, Diet RC Cola was the first product manufactured with Splenda. Although sucralose has thus far passed all safety tests and animal studies, reported adverse effects include enlarged kidney and liver.

Many people report incompatibility with most of the sugar substitutes, the major complaints being headaches and diarrhea. This is important to know when recommending suggestions for making better food and beverage choices. Diabetics have no choice but to use synthetic sweeteners. If your client is diabetic and is not amenable to using sugar substitutes, the following can be suggested as alternatives:

- Stevia (Sweet Leaf, Honey Leaf) is a plant derivative from South America. Like artificial sweeteners, stevia is not metabolized by the human body like sugar. Due to animal studies indicating stevia causes infertility, the FDA, the World Health Organization, and Canadian and European food watchdogs warn that stevia should not be used to sweeten food and beverages.[10] Currently, it is sold as a supplement and can be purchased in health food stores as an alternative to saccharine, aspartame, and sucralose.
- Sucanet is whole cane sugar with water removed.
- Fruit juice

Groups at Risk for Dental Caries

Not all clients are in need of diet counseling for dental caries, so it is important to learn to identify those groups that are most at risk: children and the elderly.[11]

Children average seven eating events in a day, most of which contain foods with added sugar. People who have more than three to five exposures per day have higher incidence of dental caries. Box 9-6 explains what constitutes an eating event.

The elderly are at risk due to xerostomia. There are two main reasons for dry mouth in the geriatric population: As we age, we lose the sense of thirst, and many elderly clients will report taking several medications, most of which manifest xerostomia. A dry mouth is one without the benefits of saliva.

BOX 9.6

EATING EVENTS

Exposures = eating a carbohydrate 20 min before or after a meal

BOX 9.7

GROUPS AT RISK FOR DENTAL CARIES

- Those with a high-carbohydrate diet
- Children/adolescents
- Elderly
- Those with past experience with dental caries
- People with xerostomia
- Those who have inadequate fluoride intake
- People with poor oral hygiene practices

Other groups at risk for dental caries are:

- anyone with past caries experience: visible caries, restorations placed within the past 3 years.
- those reporting long-term or frequent use of antihypertensive, antidepressant, antihistamine, diuretic, analgesic, and other tranquilizing drugs that decrease saliva.
- patients with diseases that contribute to dry mouth, including cancer, diabetes, anemia, salivary gland dystrophy, stroke, Alzheimer's, Sjögren's syndrome, autoimmune diseases, Parkinson's, and palsy.
- nutrition supplements, such as ma huang and ephedra, that cause dry mouth.
- people on a soft diet.
- anyone who reports eating a high-carbohydrate diet and patients who report eating frequent snacks consisting of added sugar: nibblers, grazers, or sippers of sodas and sugared coffee and tea.
- people living in an area with a nonfluoridated water supply.
- patients with visible heavy plaque and those with physical limitations that prevent thorough oral hygiene.
- young patients whose parents or caregivers have caries activity.[12]

Box 9-7 identifies groups at risk for dental caries.

A Word on Sodas

The photo in Figure 9-7 was taken of an adult who reported sipping on two to three sodas daily.

One 12-oz can of regular soda contains 10 teaspoons of sugar, give or take a few depending on the brand. According to the Academy of General Dentistry website, **noncola drinks** and **canned iced teas** are actually more harmful to enamel than Coke, Dr. Pepper, and Pepsi because flavor additives like malic and tartatic and other acids aggressively demineralize enamel. Sprite, Mountain Dew, Ginger-Ale, and Arizona Iced Tea

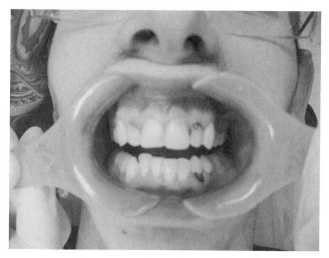

Figure 9-7. Adult soda sipper.

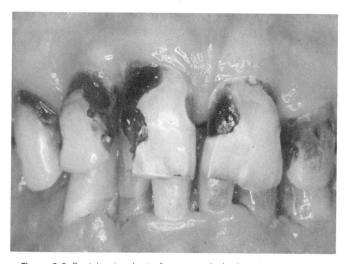

Figure 9-8. Dental caries due to frequent carbohydrate consumption.

proved to be most harmful, and root beer, brewed black tea, black coffee, and water were the least harmful to enamel.[13] A soda consumed with meals does less damage to teeth than when consumed alone or sipped throughout the day. If your patient wants to drink sodas, suggest drinking the whole can or bottle with a meal. Drinking the soda through a straw may also help reduce enamel demineralization.

Many patients report switching to diet soda to reduce the detrimental effects of regular sugared soda. They should be made aware that diet sodas have citric and phosphoric acid with a pH of 2.3 to 2.6 added as flavor enhancers, and that this acid can erode enamel and rapidly drop the pH of the oral cavity to a critical level.

Suggestions for reducing the caries potential of soda in the diet (from the Academy of General Dentistry website) include:

- Rinse the mouth with water after drinking soda to eliminate excess sugar that could be used by bacteria to make acid.
- Bypass the teeth by drinking soda from a straw.
- Drink soda from a can rather than a bottle, which can be capped and sipped throughout the day.

Counseling Patients

It is important to explain the relationship of food to disease in the oral cavity, and discuss factors that can lessen the impact of sugar in the diet. It is impractical to think that your patients will eliminate all carbohydrates from their diet and unwise to suggest eliminating any favorite food or drink. The best advice would be to rearrange the sequence of foods and beverages within meals and throughout the day. Work at raising the oral pH by including the following cariostatic foods in the diet:

- Cheese (counsel that the protective factors of cheese are lost if eaten with a cookie or cracker or followed with acidic beverage)
  - Aged cheddar
  - Swiss
  - Blue
  - Monterey Jack
  - Mozzarella
  - Brie
  - Gouda
- Peanuts
- Artificial sweeteners
- Crunchy foods
- Sugar-free chewing gum

Other good suggestions:

- If at all possible, reduce frequency of consuming sugary and acidic foods.[14,15]
- Eliminate snacking on carbohydrates before bedtime.
- Combine foods—eat sweets after proteins and fats or follow sugared foods with cheese.
- Combine raw, crunchy foods that stimulate saliva with cooked foods.
- Citrus fruits (citric acid) stimulate saliva production.
- Limit sweetened beverages to meals.[16]
- Eat cookies with milk—lactose has calcium and phosphate.

- Drink iced tea instead of soda—tea contains fluoride.[17]
- Drink orange juice with calcium to counteract the acid.[18]
- Don't rush to brush after acidic beverages—let the oral cavity remineralize enamel on its own. (Brushing may remove demineralized structure before it has a chance to remineralize.)
- Chewing sugar-free gum stimulates salivary flow that may be effective in neutralizing interproximal plaque acid through mechanical action.
- After sugared gum has lost its flavor, the chewing action can do the same thing as the sugar-free gum.
- Use a fluoridated toothpaste.[19]

PUTTING THIS INTO PRACTICE

Your client is a 23-year-old female graduate student who presents at your dental practice after a 5-year absence from professional dental care. She reports good health with use of antihistamines as needed for seasonal allergies. Radiographic and clinical exams reveal five new posterior interproximal carious lesions, and recurrent caries around two existing anterior restorations. A quick inquiry into her diet indicates high intake of carbohydrates, preference for soft foods, and frequent use of sugared breath mints. Home care consists of daily brushing for about 45 seconds and flossing two or three times per week.

1. List all factors in the above scenario that could contribute to dental caries formation, explaining in detail their relationship.
2. Write the advice you would give this client to help reduce future caries development.

CHAPTER QUIZ

1. The bacteria mainly responsible for dental caries are:
   a. Actinomycetemcomitans and *Lactobacillus*
   b. *Streptococcus mutans* and *Bacteroides forsythus*
   c. *Lactobacillus* and *Streptococcus mutans*
   d. *Streptococcus mutans* and *Streptococcus sanguis*

2. One of the components in saliva that increases the pH level in the oral cavity is:
   a. Calcium
   b. Sodium bicarbonate
   c. Phosphorus
   d. Lactic acid
   e. SLPI protein

3. Salivary fluoride levels are elevated after brushing with a fluoridated dentifrice for about:
   a. 1/4 hour
   b. 1/2 hour
   c. 1 hour
   d. 2 hours
   e. 3 hours

4. The most abundant acid produced by bacterial metabolism of carbohydrates is:
   a. Lactic
   b. Proprionic
   c. Butyric
   d. Acetic
   e. Formic

5. All foods and beverages that contain carbohydrates have the potential to cause dental caries.
   a. True
   b. False

6. The presence of calcium and phosphorus in saliva can increase the pH of the oral cavity.
   a. True
   b. False

7. The most important factor about sugar's relationship to dental caries is:
   a. Frequency of ingestion
   b. Amount of ingestion
   c. Whether it is solid or liquid
   d. Whether it is intrinsic or extrinsic

8. Which of the following would take longer to clear from the oral cavity?

   a. Cracker

   b. Ice cream

   c. Hard candy

   d. Soda

   e. Pudding

9. Which of the following sugar alcohols is the best sugar substitute due to its nonacidogenic properties?

   a. Sorbitol

   b. Mannitol

   c. Xylitol

   d. Maltitol

   e. Lactitol

10. Which of the following foods is NOT cariostatic?

    a. Cheese

    b. Peanuts

    c. Sugar-free chewing gum

    d. Apples

Web Resources

Academy of General Dentistry—Protecting Your Teeth from Food http://www.agd.org/consumer/topics/childrensnutrition/foodcavities.html

Academy of General Dentistry—Schools Long-Term Soda Deals Kick Kids in the Teeth http://www.agd.org/consumer/topics/childrensnutrition/soda.html

Academy of General Dentistry—Soda Attack: Soft Drinks, Especially Non-Colas and Iced Tea, Hurt Hard Enamel http://www.agd.org/media/2004/june/drinks.html

National Institute of Nutrition—The Effect of Diet on Dental Health http://www.nin.ca/public_html/Publications/NinReview/winter97.html#Decay Process

World Sugar Research Organization Information—Sugar and Dental Caries http://www.wsro.org/public/sugarandhealth/sugaranddentalcaries.html

Wrigley—Sugarfree Chewing Gum and Dental Caries Prevention http://www.wrigley.com/wrigley/products/dentalprofessionals.asp

References

1. Steffen JM. The effects of soft drinks on etched and sealed enamel. Angle Orthod. 1996;66(6):449–456.

2. Makinen KK, Isotupa KP, Kivilompolo T, Makinen PL, Toivanen J, Soderling E. Comparison of erythritol and xylitol saliva stimulants in the control of dental plaque and mutans streptococci. Caries Res. 2001;35(2):129–35.

3. Moss S. Relationship between fluoride, saliva, and diet. Dent Hyg News 1994;7(4):3–6.

4. Campus G, Lallai MR, Carboni R. Fluoride concentration in saliva after use of oral hygiene products. Caries Res. 2003;37(1):66–70.

5. Alty CT. The wonders of spit. RDH 2003:54–58.

6. Marshall TA, Levy SM, Broffitt B, Warren JJ, Eichengerger-Gilmore JM, Burns TL, Stumbo PJ. Dental caries and beverage consumption in young children. Pediatrics 2003;112(3 pt 1):e184–191.

7. Effects of sugar on oral health; review and recommendations. Dent Abstracts 2002; 47:I4.

8. Gilbert D. The University Record, News and Information Services, March 29, 1993.

9. Beiswanger BB, Boneta AE, Mau MS, Katz BP, Proskin HM, Stookey GK. The effect of chewing sugar-free gum after meals on clinical caries incidence. J Am Dent Assoc 1998;129(11):1623–1626.

10. Schardt D. Sweet nothings, not all sweeteners are equal. Nutrition Action Healthletter 2004:8–11.

11. Featherstone JD. The caries balance: contributing factors and early detection. J Calif Dent Assoc. 2003;31(2):129–133.

12. Featherstone J. Tipping the scales toward caries control. Dimens of Dent Hyg. 2004:20–27.

13. von Fraunhofer. Title of article? J Gen Dent. 2004. Available at: http://www.agd.org/library/issue.index.html. Accessed

14. Loveren C, Duggal MS. Experts' opinions on the role of diet in caries prevention. Caries Res. 2004;38 (Suppl 1):16–23.

15. Levy SM, Warren JJ, Broffitt B, Hillis SL, Kanellis MJ. Fluoride, beverages and dental caries in the primary dentition. Caries Res. 2003;37(3):157–165.

16. Mobley CC. Nutrition and dental caries. Dent Clin North Am. 2003;47(2):319–336.

17. Behrendt A, Oberste V, Wetzel WE. Fluoride concentration and pH of iced tea products. Caries Res. 2002;36(6):405–410.

18. Larsen MJ, Nuvad B. Enamel erosion by some soft drinks and orange juices relative to their pH, buffering effect and contents of calcium phosphate. Caries Res. 1999;33(1):81–87.

19. Watt RG, McClone P. Prevention part 2: dietary advice in the dental surgery. Br Dent J. 2003;195(1):27–31.

Suggested Readings

Alvarez JO. Nutrition, tooth development, and dental caries. Am J Clin Res. 1995;61:410S–416S.

Bibby BG, Mundorff SA, Zero DT, Almekinder KJ. Oral food clearance and the pH of plaque and saliva. J Am Dent Assoc. 1986;112(3):333–337.

Code of Federal Regulations, Title 21, Vol 2: U.S. Government Printing Office, April 2002.

Commonwealth Dental Association. Position paper on diet, nutrition, and the prevention of dental caries and erosion 2002. http://www.cdauk.com

Curnow MM, Pine CM, Burnside G, Nicholson JA, Chesters RK, Huntington E. A randomised controlled trial of the efficacy of supervised toothbrushing in high-caries-risk children. Caries Res. 2002;36(4):294–300.

Cury JA, Rebello MA, Del Bel Cury AA. In situ relationship between sucrose exposure and the composition of dental plaque. Caries Res. 1997;31(5):356–360.

Dong YM, Pearce EI, Yue L, Larsen MJ, Gao XJ, Wang JD. Plaque pH and associated parameters in relation to caries. Caries Res. 1999;33(6):428–436.

Duggal MS, van Loveren C. Dental considerations for dietary counseling. Int Dent J. 2001;51(Suppl 1):408–412.

Gutkowski S. Chew gum, build enamel. RDH. May 2002:37–38.

Hackett AF, Rugg-Gunn AJ, Murray JJ, Roberts GJ. Can breast feeding cause dental caries? Hum Nut Appl nutr. 1984; 38(1):23–28.

Harris NO, Garcia-Godoy F. Primary Preventive Dentistry. Upper Saddle River, NJ: Prentice Hall, 2003.

Heller KE, Burt BA, Eklund SA. Sugared soda consumption and dental caries in the United States. J Dent Res. 2001;80(10):1949–1953.

Hornick B. Diet and nutrition implications for oral health. J Dent Hyg. 2002; 76(1): 67–78.

Kashket S, DePaola DP. Cheese consumption and the development and progression of dental caries. J Int Assoc Dent Child 1990;20(1):3–7.

Linke HA, Moss SJ, Arav L, Chiu PM. Intra-oral lactic acid production during clearance of different foods containing various carbohydrates. Z Ernahungswiss 1997;36(2):191–197.

Linke HA, Riba HK. Oral clearance and acid production of dairy products during interaction with sweet foods. Ann Nutr Metab. 2001;45(5):202–208.

Luke GA, Gough H, Beeley JA, Geddes DA. Human salivary sugar clearance after sugar rinses and intake of foodstuffs. Caries Res. 1999;33(2):123–129.

Moynihan PJ. Dietary advice in dental practice. Br Dent J. 2002;193(10):563–568.

Nobre dos Santos M, Melo dos Santos L, Francisco SB, Cury JA. Relationship among dental plaque composition, daily sugar exposure and caries in the primary dentition. Caries Res. 2002;36(5):347–352.

O'Sullivan EA, Curzon, MEJ. A comparison of acidic dietary factors in children with and without dental erosion. J Dent Child 2000;67:186–192.

Palmer C. Diet and Nutrition in Oral Health. Upper Saddle River, NJ: Prentice Hall, 2003.

Pearce EI, Sissons CH, Coleman M, Wang X, Anderson SA, Wong L. The effect of sucrose application frequency and basal nutrient conditions on the calcium and phosphate content of experimental dental plaque. Caries Res. 2002;36(2):87–92.

Peressini S. Pacifier use and early childhood caries: an evidence-based study of the literature. J Can Dent Assoc. 2003;69(1):16–19.

American Academy of Pediatric Dentistry. Policy paper on early childhood caries (ECC): unique challenges and treatment options, 2003.

Shannon IL, McCartney JC. Presweetened dry breakfast cereals: potential for dental danger. ASDC J Dent Child 1981;48(3):215–218.

Sheiham A. Changing trends in dental caries. Int J Epidemiol. 1984;13(2);142–147.

Sheiham A. Dietary effects on dental disease. Public Health Nutr. 2001;4(2B): 569–591.

Tinanoff N, Palmer CA. Dietary determinants of dental caries and dietary recommendations for preschool children. J Public Health Dent. 2000;60(3):197–206.

Touger-Decker R, van Loveren C. Sugars and dental caries. J Am Clinl Nutr. 2003;78(4):881S–892S.

Woodward M, Walker AR. Sugar consumption and dental caries: evidence from 90 countries. Br Dent J. 1994;176(8):297–302.

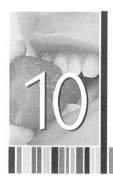

DIET, NUTRITION, AND PERIODONTAL DISEASE

Introduction

The connection of what we eat to the occurrence of dental caries is well-established, while the relationship between our diet and periodontal disease is less clear. This relationship might be summed up as: "Poor nutrition does not cause periodontal disease, but it can make an existing condition worse."

Nutrition and Periodontal Disease

If poor nutrition does not have a causal relationship with periodontal disease, at least knowing which nutrients keep the tissues healthy and which nutrients can repair diseased tissue will help us counsel patients with active periodontal disease and those at risk, steering them toward better oral health. Overall nutritional status of an individual can secondarily affect the host susceptibility and influence disease progression.[1,2]

A well-nourished host can be a primary factor in balancing the severity of periodontal disease and reducing its extent.

Periodontal disease is a bacterial infection of the periodontium. If it is limited to an inflammation of the gingival tissues, it is called gingivitis, and if it extends to periodontal ligaments, bone, and cementum, it is called periodontitis.[3] Once the bone has been affected, it is an irreversible state of disease. Figures 10-1 through 10-4 are examples of various degrees of periodontal disease.

When bacteria begin their attack on periodontal tissues, the body sends an arsenal of defense mechanisms to limit bacteria's detrimental effects and to repair the damage. A well-nourished host can offer other nutrients to help with the assault. Certain nutrients have more influence than others in building, maintaining, and repairing periodontal tissues, some with a single function and others with multiple benefits. Box 10-1 lists nutrients that assist with tissue synthesis.

All of the nutrients together will:
- build healthy soft and hard periodontal tissues
- enhance the immune system to fight infection
- regulate the immune response
- help with wound healing

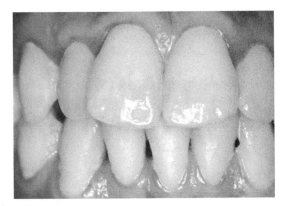

Figure 10-1. Slight plaque-induced gingivitis. Note the very early erythema (redness) of gingival margin. (From Nield-Gehrig J, Willmann D. Foundations of Periodontics for the Dental Hygienist. Baltimore: Lippincott Williams & Wilkins, 2003.)

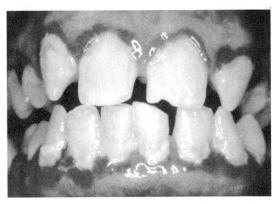

Figure 10-2. Severe plaque-induced gingivitis. Note the obvious erythema and edema of the gingival margins and papillae. (From Nield-Gehrig J, Willmann D. Foundations of Periodontics for the Dental Hygienist. Baltimore: Lippincott Williams & Wilkins, 2003.)

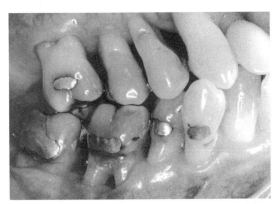

Figure 10-3. Chronic periodontitis showing blunting of the interdental papillae and gingival recession. (From Nield-Gehrig J, Willmann D. Foundations of Periodontics for the Dental Hygienist. Baltimore: Lippincott Williams & Wilkins, 2003.)

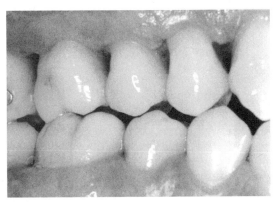

Figure 10-4. Aggressive periodontitis in a patient with good plaque control. In aggressive periodontitis, the disease severity typically seems exaggerated given the amount of bacterial plaque. (From Nield-Gehrig J, Willmann D. Foundations of Periodontics for the Dental Hygienist. Baltimore: Lippincott Williams & Wilkins, 2003.)

BOX 10.1

NUTRIENTS THAT ASSIST WITH TISSUE SYNTHESIS

- Vitamin A
- B-complex
- Vitamin D
- Calcium
- Magnesium
- Protein

Building Healthy Periodontal Tissues

Building and maintaining healthy oral tissue is the body's first line of defense against periodontal disease. Healthy oral tissue is less susceptible to infection: A strong immune system can fight off initial bacterial invasion.[2]

The epithelial lining of the gingival sulcus requires an adequate supply of nutrients because it has one of the fastest turnover rates in the body (3 days). Vitamins A, B-complex, and D and calcium and magnesium all work to build and maintain healthy soft tissue and bone.

Vitamin A assists in the formation of healthy epithelium and is vital for functioning of the immune system. If a periodontally involved patient has unhealthy pocket lining, it is usually inadvertently curettaged during deposit removal. Eating foods rich in vitamin A will assist the body in forming new healthy epithelial tissue in the sulcus. Without sufficient amounts of vitamin A, there can be an altered response to infection and the scaling site could take longer to heal.

The **B-complex vitamins**—thiamin, riboflavin, niacin, pyroxidine, cobalamin, folic acid, biotin, and pantothenic acid—are important in helping the body to form new cells and in keeping the immune system healthy. Because the B-complex vitamins are cofactors and work together, a deficiency will involve more than one.

Vitamin D enhances the absorption of calcium and magnesium, principal minerals for bone development and regeneration. Calcified tissues in the body continue to remodel throughout life, so a steady amount of these nutrients is necessary. **Calcium** and **magnesium** are principal minerals that build skeletal bones and teeth. They give strength to the alveolar bone, which is important for overall dental health. It is necessary for the alveolar process to be well-mineralized to support the structure of the teeth. With periodontal disease, bone is resorbed and teeth become loose. Decreased dietary intake of calcium results in more severe periodontal disease.[4]

Repairing Periodontal Infection

Periodontal infection is a "wound," and the body needs nutrients that will help repair tissues and convert diseased tissue to healthy tissue. Inadequate nutrition may cause impairment in the repair process of the gingival sulcus. Deficiencies of other nutrients

BOX 10.2

NUTRIENTS THAT REPAIR

- Protein
- Vitamin C
- Iron
- Zinc
- Copper
- Selenium

will cause an increase in the permeability of the epithelial attachment, which allows infection to set in. Box 10-2 lists the nutrients that repair diseased or wounded tissue.

Trace minerals are needed for protein synthesis, and **protein** supports growth and maintenance of healthy cells and plays a role in resisting infection. Antibodies are made from proteins that are targeted to destroy specific foreign particles that invade the body, whether it is a bacterium, virus, or other toxin.

Vitamin C aids in the formation of collagen, a cementing substance that helps wounds heal and assists the body's resistance to infection. It also promotes capillary integrity and enhances the body's immune response. Research shows that when compared to a group with adequate daily intake of vitamin C, those with inadequate daily intake had a higher incidence of periodontal disease.[4,5] The dietary deficiency disease of vitamin C—scurvy—will cause red, swollen, bleeding gingival tissues.

Iron, zinc, and copper assist with collagen formation and, therefore, the healing of wounds. They also perform the major function of regulating the inflammatory response.

Selenium's antioxidant qualities work to prevent harm to cells and tissues. Table 10-1 identifies all the nutrients and minerals and their function in building, maintaining, and repairing healthy periodontium.

Table 10-1. Functions of Nutrients and Minerals

Nutrient	Function	Mineral	Function
Vitamin A	• Builds and maintains healthy epithelium • Aids immune system	Calcium	• Builds and maintains strong alveolar process
B-complex	• Forms new cells • Keeps immune system healthy	Iron	• Forms collagen • Aids with wound healing • Regulates inflammatory response
Vitamin D	• Aids with calcium absorption	Zinc	• Forms collagen • Aids with wound healing • Regulates inflammatory response
Vitamin C	• Aids with wound healing • Helps the body resist infection	Copper	• Aids with wound healing
		Selenium	• Prevents harm to cells
Protein	• Promotes growth, maintenance, and repair of all body tissues	Magnesium	• Works with vitamin D and calcium to build and maintain strong alveolar bone

Dental Charting
- Class I amalgam restorations in first molars
- Porcelain crown #9
- Suspicious area occlusal #31
- Impacted third molars

Nutritional Survey Assessment
- Irregular eating habits
- Patient is a musician and is primarily nocturnal
- Meals consist of fast food and convenience microwavable meals
- Lactose intolerant
- Avoids foods with crunchy consistency due to popping in TMJ

1. Based on the assessment information, evaluate the need for nutritional counseling and explain where your time could best be spent.

2. Outline the source of his nutrient deficiency based on the information given regarding his eating habits.

3. List some ideal foods with specific nutrients and state why the food/nutrient is needed in his diet.

4. Based on your suggestions, what do you expect in the way of improvement of periodontal health?

CHAPTER QUIZ

1. The physical consistency of food is important to periodontal structures because:

   a. Plaque can be removed at the gingival 1/3 when eating crunchy foods

   b. The act of chewing crunchy foods brings saliva into the mouth for antibacterial effects

   c. Soft foods clear the oral cavity faster than hard foods

   d. Hard, crunchy foods strengthen keratinized tissues

2. Nutrients that have an effect on wound healing are:

   a. Vitamin C and zinc

   b. Selenium and magnesium

   c. Vitamin D and calcium

   d. Vitamin A and B-complex

3. Nutritional recommendations for maintaining healthy oral tissues should include:

   a. Taking double the RDA for vitamin C

   b. Increasing dairy products and limiting carbohydrates

   c. Taking a multivitamin and following the Food Guide Pyramid

   d. Limiting hard, crunchy foods to only one per day

4. Healthy oral tissues are the body's first line of defense against periodontal disease.

   a. True

   b. False

5. Poor nutrition is the initiating factor in periodontal disease.

   a. True

   b. False

Web Resources

American Academy of Periodontology
www.perio.org

UCLA Periodontics Information Center
http://www.dent.ucla.edu/pic/links.html

References

1. Position paper on periodontal disease as a potential risk factor for systemic diseases. J Periodontol. 2000;69:841–850.

2. Boyd LD, Madden TE. Nutrition, infection, and periodontal disease. Dent Clin North Am. 2003;47(2): 337–354.

3. Gehrig J, Willmann D. Foundations of Periodontics for the Dental Hygienist. Baltimore: Lippincott Williams and Wilkins, 2003.

4. Nishida M, Grossi SG, Dunford RG, Ho AW, Trevisan M, Genco RJ. Calcium and the risk for periodontal disease. J Periondontol. 2000;71(7): 1057–1066.

5. Nishida M, Grossi SG, Dunford RG, Ho AW, Trevisan M, Genco RJ. Dietary vitamin C and the risk for periodontal disease. J Periodontol. 2000;71(8):1215–1223.

6. Lowe G, Woodward M, Rumley A, Morrison C, Tunstall-Pedoe H, Stephen K. Total tooth loss and prevalent cardiovascular disease in men and women: possible roles of citrus fruit consumption, vitamin C, and inflammatory and thrombotic variables. J Clin Epidemiol. 2003;56 (7):694–700.

Suggested Readings

Boyd LD, Lampi KJ. Importance of nutrition for optimum health of the periodontium. J Contemp Dent Pract. 2001;2 (2):36–45.

Carranza FA, Newman MG. Clinical Periodontology. Influence of Systemic Diseases on the Periodontium. Philadelphia: W. B. Saunders, 1996.

Davis JR, Stegeman CA. The Dental Hygienist's Guide to Nutritional Care. Philadelphia: W. B. Saunders, 1998.

Genco RJ, Goldman, HM, Cohen DW. Contemporary Periodontics. St. Louis: Mosby, 1990.

Mobley C, Dodds M. Diet, nutrition and teeth. In: Palmer CA, ed. Diet and Nutrition in Oral Health. Upper Saddle River, NJ: Prentice Hall 2003.

Nevia RF, Steigenga J, Al-Shammari KF, Wang HL. Effects of specific nutrients on periodontal disease onset, progression and treatment. J Clin Periodontol. 2003; 30(7):579–589.

Nizel AE, Papas AS. Nutrition in Clinical Dentistry. Philadelphia: W. B. Saunders, 1989.

Position paper on diabetes and periodontal diseases. J Periodontol. 2000;71:664–678.

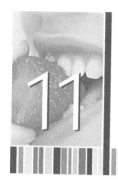

CHOOSING FOODS WISELY

Introduction

How do you know if you are choosing foods wisely to maintain good health and keep you disease-free? What is a long healthy life worth to you? The amount of nutrition information is daunting, some of it credible and some not completely accurate. How do you filter through the information to choose what is best for your family while enjoying the process of preparing and eating tasty meals? The answer is to follow guidelines developed by credible sources with proven track records that will lead us through life, healthy and disease-free. Most countries have developed plans for good nutrition that include guidelines and pictorial representations as suggestions to help maintain health. Following established dietary guidelines, making our food selections according to a healthy food graphic, and utilizing good food-handling and safety measures ensure a course for better health and possibly a longer life.

Dietary Guidelines

The *Dietary Guidelines for Americans* made its debut in 1980, and is updated, by law, every 5 years (the 2005 *Dietary Guidelines* are available at http://www.health.gov/dietaryguidelines). The purpose of the publication is to help Americans choose a balanced, healthy diet. The guidelines are used to set standards for federal nutrition programs such as school lunch programs, and if followed, have a great impact on the foods we choose to buy. Other countries have established their own guidelines, taking into account cultural preferences and seasonal availability of certain foods. Because we live in a globally connected world, many of our clients may be following a different set of guidelines. Reading other countries' nutritional guidelines emphasizes the fact that the intended use for all is to keep people healthy. The following is a sampling of dietary guidelines from around the world, many with similar messages as the United States, and all with good advice that is helpful wherever you live.

Australia

- Enjoy a wide variety of nutritious foods.
- Eat plenty of vegetables, legumes, and fruits.
- Eat plenty of cereals (including breads, rice, pasta, and noodles), preferably whole grain.
- Include lean meat, fish, poultry, and/or alternatives.
- Include milks, yogurts, cheeses, and/or alternatives. Reduced-fat varieties should be chosen, where possible.
- Drink plenty of water.

Take care to:

- limit saturated fat and moderate total fat intake.
- choose foods low in salt.
- limit your alcohol intake if you choose to drink.
- consume only moderate amounts of sugars and foods containing added sugars.
- prevent weight gain: be physically active and eat according to your energy needs.
- care for your food: prepare and store it safely.
- encourage and support breastfeeding.

Canada

- Enjoy a variety of foods.
- Emphasize cereals, breads, other grain products, vegetables, and fruits.
- Choose lower-fat dairy products, leaner meats, and food prepared with little or no fat.
- Achieve and maintain a healthy body weight by enjoying regular physical activity and healthy eating.
- Limit salt, alcohol, and caffeine.

Germany

- Choose from among many different foods.
- Eat cereal products several times per day and plenty of potatoes.
- Eat fruits and vegetables often—take "5 a day."
- Consume milk and dairy products daily, fish once a week, and meat, sausages, and eggs in moderation.
- Restrict dietary fat to 70 to 90 g/day, preferably of plant origin.
- Use sugar and salt in moderation—be creative in using herbs and spices.
- Drink plenty of liquids—water is vitally necessary. Drink alcohol in moderation.
- Make sure your dishes are prepared gently and taste well.
- Take your time and enjoy eating.
- Watch your weight and stay active.

Great Britain

- Enjoy your food.
- Eat a variety of different foods.
- Eat the right amount to be a healthy weight—energy needs are dependent on gender, age, body size, and activity level.
- Eat plenty of foods rich in starch and fiber.
- Eat plenty of fruits and vegetables.
- Don't eat too many foods that contain a lot of fat.
- Don't have sugary foods and drinks too often.
- Don't eat too many foods high in salt, and cut down on the amount of salt added in cooking and at the table.

India

- Overall energy intake should be restricted to levels commensurate to the sedentary occupations of the affluent, so obesity is avoided.
- Highly refined and polished cereals should be avoided in preference to under-milled cereals.
- Green leafy vegetables (a source not only of carotene but also of linolenic acid derivatives) should be included at least in levels recommended by International Conference on Dietary Guidelines.
- Edible fat intake need not exceed 40 g, and total fat intake should be limited to levels at which fat will provide no more than 20% of total energy. The use of clarified butter should be restricted for special occasions and should not be a regular daily feature.
- Intake of sugar and sweets should be restricted.
- High salt intake should be restricted.

Ireland

- Enjoy your food.
- Eat a variety of different foods, using the Food Pyramid as a guide.
- Eat the right amount of food to be a healthy weight, and exercise regularly. Foods with a lot of fiber fill you up quickly, so you'll be less likely to want high-fat foods. This will help you be a healthy weight.
- Eat four or more portions of fruit and vegetables every day. Try to get into the habit of having at least one portion of fruit juice, fruit, or vegetable at each meal.
- Eat more foods rich in starch—breads and cereals (especially whole grain), potatoes, pasta and rice, and fruit and vegetables.
- Reduce the amount of fatty foods you eat, especially saturated fats. Make lower fat choices whenever possible. Grill, boil, oven-bake, or stir-fry in very little fat instead of deep-frying. Try eating fewer foods from the top of the Food Pyramid.

- If you drink alcohol, keep within sensible limits. Preferably, drink with meals and try to make every second day an alcohol-free day.
- Use a variety of seasonings; try not to always rely on salt to flavor foods. Use herbs, spices, and black pepper as alternatives.
- If you drink or eat snacks containing sugar, limit the number of times you take them throughout the day. This is particularly important for children's growing teeth.

Korea

- Eat a variety of foods.
- Maintain your ideal body weight.
- Eat sufficient amounts of protein.
- Eat 20% total energy intake from fats.
- Drink milk every day.
- Choose a diet low in salt.
- Maintain your teeth's health.
- Restrict smoking and drinking of alcohol and caffeinated beverages.
- Maintain a balance between energy intake and expenditure.
- Enjoy homemade meals to be happy with families.

Philippines

- Eat a variety of foods every day. (Eat a balanced diet from a variety of foods; pay particular attention to your food needs during pregnancy and lactation; prepare meals for your children that are varied, complete, and adequate for their growth and development; support the elderly with a diet suitable to their conditions; choose ready-to-eat foods with high nutritional value.)
- Promote breastfeeding and proper weaning. (Learn about and promote the advantages and value of breastfeeding; learn the techniques of successful breast-feeding; breastfeed for as long as there is milk; start supplementary foods when the baby is 4 to 6 months old.)
- Achieve and maintain desirable body weight. (Weigh yourself and the members of your family regularly and behave accordingly; maintain energy balance to desirable body weight; exercise regularly—it's good for you.)
- Eat clean and safe food. (Learn to prevent food-borne diseases; practice safe food storage, handling, preparation, and service.)
- Practice a healthy lifestyle. (Be moderate in what you eat and drink; avoid smoking and control stress; maintain good dental health.)

United States

- Aim for a healthy weight.
- Be physically active each day.
- Let the Food Pyramid guide your food choices.
- Choose a variety of grains daily, especially whole grains.
- Choose a variety of fruits and vegetables daily.
- Keep food safe to eat.
- Choose a diet that is low in saturated fat and cholesterol and moderate in total fat.
- Choose beverages and food to moderate intake of sugars.
- Choose and prepare foods with less salt.
- If you drink alcoholic beverages, do so in moderation.

Unified Dietary Guidelines

Before 1999, major health organizations for cancer, heart disease, diabetes, and hypertension each had their own set of dietary guidelines for people to follow to reduce their risk of certain diseases. It is not unusual for a person to have more than one disease, such as the combination of diabetes and heart disease or having hypertension and hypercholesteremia. Having several guidelines to follow is confusing, and oftentimes they fall by the wayside. To help with compliance, the organizations united their suggestions and developed one set of guidelines for healthy eating—the Unified Dietary Guidelines. The Unified Dietary Guidelines have been approved by the American Cancer Society, American Heart Association, American Dietetic Association, American Academy of Pediatrics, and National Institute of Health, and if followed, will reduce the risk for many chronic diseases. The following is a list of their suggestions:

- Eat a variety of foods; choose most of what you eat from plant sources.
- Eat six or more servings of breads, cereals, pasta, and grains each day.
- Choose five or more servings of vegetables per day.
- Eat high-fat foods sparingly, especially those from animal sources. Choose fats and oils with 2 g or less saturated fat per tablespoon, such as liquid and tub margarines, canola oil, and olive oil.
- Keep your intake of simple sugars to a minimum.
- Balance the number of calories you eat with the number you use each day.
- Eat less than 6 g of salt (sodium chloride) per day (2,400 milligrams of sodium).
- Have no more than one alcoholic drink per day if you're a woman and no more than two if you're a man.

DISTINGUISHING FRUITS AND VEGETABLES

Fruits contain seeds.
Vegetables are plants that do not contain seeds.

5-A-Day Program

Even with the major health organizations recommending the "5-A-Day" program for fruits and vegetables, Americans consume less than three servings a day. Box 11-1 contains useful information for distinguishing fruits and vegetables. Unless fruit and vegetable dishes are dripping in butter or sugar, they are considered an excellent low-fat source of vitamins, minerals, and fiber. Avocados, coconut, and olives are the exception because they are high in fat. The National Cancer Institute (branch of the National Institutes of Health) refers to fruit and vegetables as the original "fast food." Grapes, cherry tomatoes, and bananas can be eaten on the spot without any preparation.

Any fruit or vegetable "counts" toward the goal of five a day, but knowing which are rich in vitamins A and C as well those that are considered "cruciferous" will help in choosing a good variety. The National Cancer Institute recommends choosing one fruit or vegetable high in vitamin A and one high in vitamin C per day, and several cruciferous vegetables each week to guard against certain cancers. Boxes 11-2 and 11-3 identify cruciferous vegetables and those fruits and vegetable considered good sources of fiber. Table 11-1 indicates source of vitamins A and C in fruits and vegetables.

Fresh, frozen, canned, or dried fruits and vegetables all provide vitamins, minerals, and fiber; fruit and vegetable juice also provide vitamins and minerals. A wise shopper, however, knows it makes a difference as to what form of fruit or vegetable is bought. Food is freshest if picked ripe off the vine and eaten immediately. If picked unripe, it may not contain all the nutrients. Many fruits and vegetables are harvested too early and then sprayed to retard spoilage as they travel to the grocery store and sit on the produce shelf until someone buys them. Frozen is the next best to fresh. When choosing produce from the frozen food section, shake the bag to make sure the contents move around. If the contents do not move around and the bag is one big block of ice, this indicates that the contents have been allowed to thaw, which causes the nutrients to leach out of the food

CRUCIFEROUS VEGETABLES

- Bok choy
- Broccoli
- Brussel sprouts
- Cabbage
- Cauliflower

GOOD SOURCES OF FIBER

- Apples
- Bananas
- Blackberries/blueberries/raspberries/strawberries
- Brussel sprouts
- Carrots
- Cherries
- Cooked beans and peas
- Dates/figs
- Grapefruits/oranges
- Kiwi
- Pears
- Prunes
- Spinach
- Sweet potatoes

and into the water. When refrozen, the nutrients are in the block of ice instead of in the vegetables themselves. Canned is the least desirable, as the canning process requires intense heat, which can destroy many of the B vitamins.

Food Guide Pyramids

The Food Pyramid, developed by the United States Department of Agriculture (USDA) about 14 years ago, was lauded by many to be a stroke of genius; foods to be consumed least were at the top and foods to be consumed most were spread out at the bottom. It was a simple, easy-to-understand pictorial graphic that soon adorned the sides and backs of most food packages. It didn't take long for critics to realize that basic ideas were missing. There was no mention of physical activity, water consumption, or that cereals and grains were supposed to be complex versus simple carbohydrates. All meats were lumped together without mentioning that some were leaner than others. And although fats were one of the limiting categories at the top, it failed to depict that some fats are actually desirable to have in the daily diet. The USDA has organized a panel of scientists to revamp our current Food Pyramid to help downsize our growing obese population. It should be available to consumers sometime in 2005. Figure 11-1 shows the current U.S. Food Pyramid.

Important topics to consider when interpreting the Food Pyramid are as follows:

- A healthy diet should be combined with exercise and weight control.
- Eat whole grains versus refined at most meals for satiety and more stable blood glucose levels.
- Include good sources of unsaturated fats in your daily diet, such as olive, canola,

Table 11-1.

Good source of Vitamin	A	C
Acorn squash	X	
Apricots	X	X
Bell peppers		X
Broccoli		X
Brussel sprouts		X
Cabbage		X
Cantaloupe	X	X
Carrots	X	
Cauliflower		X
Chili peppers		X
Collards	X	X
Grapefruit		X
Honeydew melon		X
Kale	X	
Kiwi		X
Leaf lettuce	X	
Mangos	X	X
Mustard greens	X	X
Oranges		X
Pineapple		X
Plums		X
Potato with skin		X
Pumpkin	X	
Romaine lettuce	X	
Spinach	X	X
Strawberries		X
Sweet potatoes	X	
Tangerines		X
Tomatoes		X
Watermelon		X
Winter squash	X	

and other vegetable oils and fatty fish such as salmon, to lower cholesterol and offer protective factors for the heart.

- Eat a variety of fresh fruit and vegetables throughout the week.
- Choose fish, poultry, eggs, nuts, and legumes as a source of protein over fatty meats such as beef and pork.
- Choose low-fat dairy products or take a calcium supplement daily.
- Eat red meat, pork, and butter sparingly.

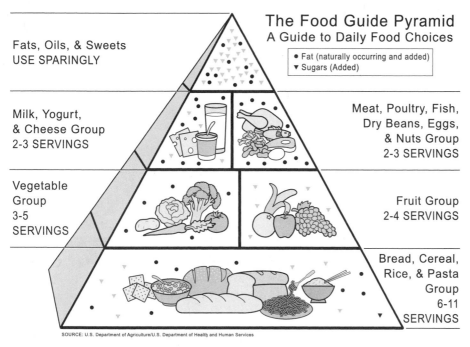

Figure 11-1. The Food Guide Pyramid.

- Eat refined and simple carbohydrates such as white rice, white bread, pasta, potatoes, and sweets sparingly.
- Take a multivitamin/mineral supplement as a back-up.
- Drink alcohol in moderation: one to two drinks per day for males and less than one drink per day for females.

Because the U.S. Food Pyramid is based on a 2,000-calorie diet for Americans, different age groups and those with differing activity levels should alter the recommendations to fit their needs. Children have different food preferences and require fewer calories. Those with a sedentary lifestyle require fewer calories than those who are in a state of growth or are very active. The serving-size suggestions for each food group are given in a range, so inactive or small people should use the lower end and the very active should use the upper range.

Other countries have developed their own pyramid or other shaped food guide that takes into consideration the country's main staple, availability of foods, and cultural preferences.

Figure 11-2 is an example of how the U.S. Food Pyramid can be adapted to meet specific dietary needs.

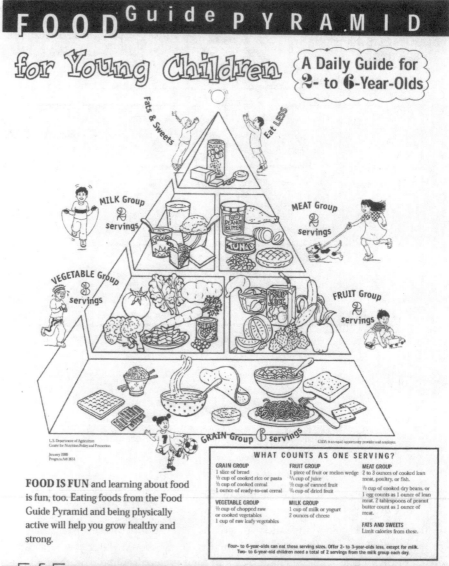

FOOD IS FUN and learning about food is fun, too. Eating foods from the Food Guide Pyramid and being physically active will help you grow healthy and strong.

Figure 11-2. The Food Guide Pyramid for Young Children. (Published in the public domain by the U.S. Department of Agriculture.)

Balancing Diet and Physical Activity

In 1993, the National Weight Control Registry was created to keep track of and identify the habits of individuals who were successful in losing and maintaining weight. Over 3,000 individuals are now in the database, making it one of the largest studies of its kind. Years of research reveal why these individuals were successful in losing at least 30 pounds and maintaining the loss for at least a year: They were highly motivated and had increased their daily physical activity level. Weight loss wasn't necessarily a result of the foods they chose or excluded from their diets. Physical activity and a sensible diet work together for better health.

Energy balance is when calories consumed are adequate for maintenance or growth. When there is an excess of calories consumed—more than needed for maintenance—weight increases. A decrease in calories results in weight loss. Weight gain or loss is referred to as energy imbalance. We need to eat each day to provide our bodies with energy to keep our hearts beating, lungs expanding, liver and kidneys filtering waste, and sodium pumps maintaining water balance. Energy (calories) is delivered to all parts of our bodies from metabolism of carbohydrates, protein, fat, and alcohol. The energy our body needs just to stay alive accounts for two-thirds of all energy spent throughout the day, leaving one-third for our physical activity. For some, there are more calories left to spend than are spent, which causes unnecessary weight gain.

Obesity is now considered to be of epidemic proportions in the United States for all age groups, and is the second major cause of death. Decreased activity levels as well as increased portion sizes have swelled our waists and given us heart disease, hypertension, stroke, certain kinds of cancer, and diabetes. What we eat and whether we exercise are both important choices to make. Hours spent surfing the Internet, watching television, and playing video games create overweight, sedentary people. Being aware of activity levels and rethinking ways to incorporate physical activity into daily routines prevent the downward spiral into obesity and its accompanying diseases. It takes a conscious effort to keep a healthy weight, keeping track of calories in and calories out. If the number of calories consumed consistently exceeds the number spent, weight increases. If you expend 3,500 more calories each week than you take in, you will lose a pound. Over time, that adds up.

The recommended 30 minutes of physical activity per day does not have to be accomplished all at once. Short bursts of activity throughout the day are also acceptable, although sustained activity levels are best for weight loss. If exercise has not been part of your daily routine, remember to start out slow and gradually build up. Starting out fast and furious can only lead to pain and injury. Box 11-4 offers suggestions on weight loss.

BOX 11.4

SUGGESTIONS ON WEIGHT LOSS

Aim for slow weight loss versus rapid weight loss.
Stay away from diets that promise rapid results.
Reducing your *weekly* diet by 3,500 calories will result in a 1-pound weight loss.

All types of physical activity are beneficial. Aerobic exercise speeds up your heart rate and breathing, keeping the circulatory system strong. Strength training, such as lifting weights, helps maintain bone strength and prevent osteoporosis. Stretching, as is done in dancing or yoga, can increase flexibility, making other activities more enjoyable. The following are examples of moderate exercise that can burn 100 to 200 extra calories per day:

- Washing and waxing a car for 45 minutes
- Gardening for 45 minutes
- Raking leaves for 30 minutes
- Walking a 15-minute mile for 30 minutes
- Pushing a baby stroller for 30 minutes
- Shooting baskets for 30 minutes
- Riding a bike for 30 minutes
- Swimming laps for 20 minutes

Figure 11-3 details the time needed to burn 200 kilocalories.
Other suggestions to incorporate physical activity into your day include:

- Limit time spent in front of the TV or computer and spend the time moving your body.
- Always opt for the stairs versus elevators or escalators.
- Ride the exercise bike as you watch TV.
- Play your favorite music and dance.
- Make the kids go outside to play instead of sitting in front of the TV or computer.
- Trade the sit-down lawnmower for the push mower.

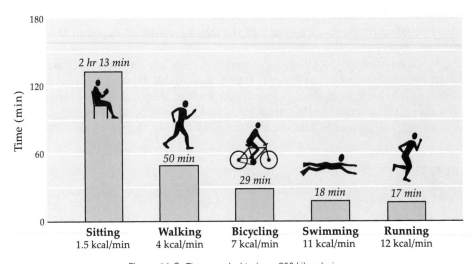

Figure 11-3. Time needed to burn 200 kilocalories.

- Park as far away from work, mall, or arena entrances as you can, and while doing so, think about how fortunate you are to be healthy enough to walk the distance.
- If at all possible, let the kids ride their bikes to school or sports practice once a week.
- Form a walking group in your neighborhood and establish a specific meeting time and place.
- Conduct a walking meeting instead of sitting around a conference table.
- Walk with coworkers to a restaurant for lunch.

Food Safety and Preparation

Even though your kitchen may rival that of an interior showplace, it may not be fit for cooking. Clean floors, spotless countertops, and organized cupboards are not indicators of a kitchen that employs "safe practices." We are unable to see, feel, or smell bacteria that contaminate our food. Keeping food safe for consumption depends on how it is stored, handled, and cooked. Eating food that contains harmful bacteria, toxins, parasites, viruses, or chemical contaminants can causes food-borne illness.

Campylobacter, Salmonella, Listeria, and *Escherichia coli* are the most common invaders. You don't have to eat a lot of contaminated food before you feel ill—you can become sick by eating just a few bites. Because food-borne illnesses resemble the common flu, many people are unaware it was the food that made them sick. Symptoms can appear about 30 minutes after eating or can take up to 3 weeks to manifest. It is estimated that up to 33 million people in the United States are sickened each year with a food-borne illness. To ensure that you are not part of this statistic, follow these four simple steps when handling or preparing food, which are highlighted in Box 11-5:

1. Clean

    a. Wash your hands for 20 seconds with hot, soapy water before and after handling food and after using the bathroom, playing with your pet, or changing diapers.

    b. Wash cutting boards, dishes, utensils, and countertops with hot, soapy water each time you prepare a new food for the meal. Box 11-6 gives advice for handling cutting boards.

BOX 11.5   **FOUR STEPS OF FOOD SAFETY**

1. Clean
2. Separate
3. Cook
4. Chill

CUTTING BOARD TIPS

- Use smooth cutting boards made of hard wood or plastic.
- Use one board for cutting meats and one for ready-to-eat foods such as vegetables, fruits, and bread.
- Boards should be free of cracks and crevices.
- Scrub boards with a brush in hot soapy water after use.
- Sanitize boards in the dishwasher or rinse in a solution of 1 teaspoon bleach in 1 quart of water.

BOX 11.6

    c. Use disposable paper towels versus cloth towels, which can harbor bacteria.

    d. Clean liquids that spill in the refrigerator, including those that leak out of packaged lunchmeat and hot dogs.

2. Separate (don't cross-contaminate)

    a. Separate raw meat, poultry, and seafood from other foods in your shopping cart and refrigerator and on the counter.

    b. Designate separate cutting boards for food groups: one for cutting meat, another for chopping vegetables, and another for slicing bread.

    c. Wash anything that comes into contact with raw meats and their juices with hot, soapy water.

    d. Use one plate for raw meat, poultry, and seafood and another plate after they are cooked.

3. Cook

    a. Use a thermometer to determine that food is fully cooked.

    b. Cook roasts and steaks to 145°, poultry to 180°, and pork to 160°.

    c. Fish is done when it flakes with a fork.

    d. Never use or eat ground beef that is still pink.

    e. Cook eggs until both the yolk and white are firm, and avoid recipes that call for raw eggs. Box 11-7 provide further egg safety tips.

    f. Microwaved food should be hot throughout with no cold spots.

    g. Reheated food should be cooked to 165° or boiled.

EGG SAFETY TIPS

- Commercial products are made with pasteurized eggs that have been heated sufficiently to kill bacteria, or they contain an acidifying agent that kills bacteria.
- Commercial cookie dough is safe to eat uncooked.
- Buy only refrigerated eggs and keep them cold until ready to cook or serve.
- Cook eggs until they no longer run or scramble eggs until there is no visible liquid.

BOX 11.7

4. Chill
   a. Keep the temperature of your refrigerator at or below 41° to slow the growth of bacteria.
   b. Refrigerate or freeze perishables, cooked food, and all leftovers within 2 hours and put a date on the container. Leftovers should be used within 3 to 5 days.
   c. Thaw food in the refrigerator, under cold water, or in the microwave—never on a counter at room temperature.
   d. Marinate all food in the refrigerator.
   e. Store leftovers in small shallow containers versus large containers for quick cooling.
   f. Don't overpack the refrigerator—cool air must circulate to keep food safe.

Figure 11-4 illustrates safe refrigeration temperatures and the danger zone for food.

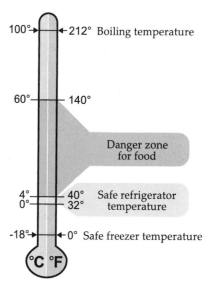

Figure 11-4. Safe refrigerator and freezer temperatures.

Other Kitchen Dangers

Other kitchen dangers include lead, microwave packaging, and insects and dirt:

- Lead leached from ceramic dishes into food and drink is the number one source of dietary lead. To reduce your exposure to lead, don't use ceramic or lead crystal containers to store food. Use them sparingly for serving.
- Microwaving can cause adhesives and polymers from the package to leach into food. If at all possible, don't use the package carton to heat your food; rather, use a microwave-safe dish.
- Wash the tops of cans before removing lids to eliminate dust and dirt from falling into the food.
- Avoid storing food in cupboards under the sink or where water can leak or drain. Insects and rodents are attracted to dark, damp places and can invade openings in packages. Box 11-8 highlights safe kitchen tips.

BOX 11.8

TIPS FOR KEEPING A SAFE KITCHEN

- Keep dishcloths and sponges clean and dry. When wet, they harbor bacteria and promote bacterial growth.
- When washing dishes by hand, wash within 2 hours and air-dry so they are not handled when wet.
- If you have an infection or cut on your hands, wear rubber gloves and wash the gloves as often as bare hands.
- When thawing food in cold water, seal it in a water-tight bag and submerge it in water, changing the water every 30 minutes.
- Food defrosted in the microwave should be cooked immediately.
- Don't buy frozen seafood if the package is open, torn, or crushed on the edges.

Counseling Patients

Sticking to the tried-and-true food guidelines are best when recommending a starting place for changing how your patient eats. Just as it is recommended that dental professionals only recommend products approved by the American Dental Association, we should suggest behaviors recommended by the Food Guidelines for Americans and the USDA Food Pyramid (or those from the patient's homeland). After collecting data and analyzing a food diary, do the following:

1. Compare the patient's food diary to suggestions made by the Food Pyramid or other food guide that would be best suited to his or her cultural considerations, and point out excesses and deficiencies.

2. Choose food guidelines best suited to your patient's medical and cultural tendencies, and suggest ways to improve in areas of neglect.

3. Recommend 30 minutes of moderate exercise each day, and work with your patient to discover ways to incorporate more movement into the daily schedule.

4. Outline safe food handling and preparation techniques to ensure your patient is keeping food safe to prevent food-borne illnesses.

PUTTING THIS INTO PRACTICE

1. Using the guidelines from around the world as examples, invent a 10-point dietary guidelines to guide your family to a healthy lifestyle.

2. Explain the key differences between the current U.S. Food Pyramid and the pyramid plus changes in the making.

3. Make a food pyramid or (other shape) to illustrate your family's current eating habits.

4. Using your family's food pyramid, list some changes that should be made to follow the dietary guidelines you invented for your family.

CHAPTER QUIZ

1. The U.S. Dietary Guidelines are updated by law every _____ year(s).
   a. 1
   b. 3
   c. 5
   d. 10

2. The Unified Dietary Guidelines are meant to replace the U.S. Dietary Guidelines and to be used by people with a diagnosed disease.
   a. True
   b. False

3. Which of the following are examples of cruciferous vegetables?
   a. Cabbage and Brussel sprouts
   b. Kidney beans and corn
   c. Leaf lettuce and cucumbers
   d. Onions and garlic

4. Which of the following country's food guidelines recommends deep-frying?
   a. Great Britain
   b. India
   c. Ireland
   d. Phillipines
   e. None of the above

5. The U.S. Food Pyramid specifically suggests eating unrefined breads, cereals, and grains.
   a. True
   b. False

6. If someone keeps a spotless kitchen, it is probably safe to eat any food dish prepared in it.
   a. True
   b. False

7. The best place to thaw meat is:
   a. On the counter at room temperature
   b. In a sealed bag submerged in cold water
   c. On a shelf under the freezer section in the refrigerator
   d. b or c
   e. Any of the above

8. It is recommended that to ensure there will be no cross-contamination, the cutting board should be cleaned of all meat juice with hot, soapy water before using it to chop vegetables.

   a. True

   b. False

9. What is the best temperature for retarding bacterial growth in the refrigerator?

   a. Under 50°

   b. Under 40°

   c. 32°

   d. 0°

10. To maintain a healthy weight, it is recommended that we get 30 minutes of sustained aerobic exercise.

    a. True

    b. False

Web Resources

Partnership for Food Safety Education—Fight Bac!: Keep Food Safe From Bacteria www.fightbac.org

Food Safety—Gateway to Government Food Safety Information www.foodsafety.gov

U.S. Food and Drug Administration—Center for Food Safety and Applied Nutrition http://vm.cfsan.fda.gov/

U.S. Food and Drug Administration www.fda.gov

U.S. Department of Health and Human Services—The Surgeon General's Call to Action to Prevent and Decrease Overweight and Obesity www.surgeon general.gov/topics/obesity

Harvard School of Public Health—Food Pyramids www.hsph.harvard.edu/nutritionsource/pyramids.html

Food Pyramid for Kids and Adults www.pediatrics.about.com

American Dietetic Association www.eatright.org

Federal Citizen Information Center www.pueblo.gsa.gov

Vegetarian Food Pyramid www.vegsource.com/nutrition/pyramid.htm

U.S. Department of Agriculture—Food Guide Pyramids www.usda.gov/news/usdakids/food_pyr.html

Food and Nutrition Information Center www.nal.usda.gov/fnic/Fpyr/pyramid.html

The British Dietetic Association http://cgi.www.bda.uk.com/

For more information about safe food handling and preparation:
1. USDA's Meat and Poultry Hotline: 1-800-535–4555
2. FDA's Food Information and Seafood Hotline: 1-800-332–4010

References

Burros M. U.S. diet proposals reflect nation's lack of fitness. New York Times, September 10, 2003.

Food Safety and Inspection Service, U.S. Department of Agriculture. Listerosis and Food Safety Tips. Washington, D.C., 1999.

Food Safety and Inspection Service, U.S. Department of Agriculture. Fight BAC! Washington, D.C.: Author

Kurtzweil P. Can your kitchen pass the food safety test? FDA Consumer Magazine, September 1998.

Kurtzweil P. Fruits and vegetables—eating your way to 5 a day. FDA Consumer Magazine, April 1999.

Painter J, Rah JH, Lee YK. Comparison of international food guide pictorial representations. J Am Dietetic Assoc. 2002;102 (4): 483–489.

Palmer CA. Diet and Nutrition in Oral Health. Upper Saddle River, NJ: Prentice Hall, 2003.

U.S. Department of Agriculture. Nutrition and your health: dietary guidelines for Americans. 5th Ed. Washington, D.C., 2000.

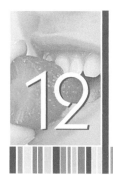

READING LABELS

Introduction

Learning to read a food label is like learning a specialized lingo. Just as you had to learn "dental speak," you also have to learn "nutrition speak." In 1990, the U.S. Food and Drug Administration (FDA) established the Nutrition Labeling and Education Act (NLEA) to help consumers know what they are buying so that they can make healthier food and snack selections. The NLEA requires food package labels for all food except meat and poultry, and is voluntary for raw produce and fish. The NLEA also set guidelines for stating nutrient claims, such as "low-fat" or "sugar-free," and certain FDA-approved health claims, such as "lowers cholesterol." All food labels are titled "Nutrition Facts" and contain the same information, allowing consumers to compare similar products and to calculate the amount of nutrients consumed daily. In 1994, food package labeling became law. The following foods are exceptions to that law and do not require food labels:

- Food served in hospital cafeterias, on airplanes, in vending machines, and at mall counters
- Bakery, deli, or candy store that serves ready-to-eat food prepared on site
- Food shipped in bulk
- Medical foods that are consumed to address the needs of certain diseases
- Coffee, tea, spices, or other nonnutritive foods
- Food served in restaurants, unless they make a health or nutrient claim on their menu, advertisement, or other notice

An American Dietetics Association survey revealed that 71% of Americans read labels, but that most become confused while doing so. Learning to separate fact from fiction is necessary to accurately read a label and to make good choices when purchasing food. Although labels are not meant to be tricky, they can be misleading if not read carefully.

Reading a Nutrition Facts Label

"Nutrition Facts" contain several parts and under the NLEA, food manufacturers are *required* to provide daily values, based on a 2,000-calorie diet, for the following:

- Total calories
- Calories from fat
- Calories from saturated fat
- Total fat
- Polyunsaturated fat
- Saturated fat
- Monounsaturated fat
- Cholesterol
- Sodium
- Potassium
- Total carbohydrate
- Dietary fiber
- Soluble fiber
- Insoluble fibers
- Sugars
- Sugar alcohols
- Protein
- Vitamin A
- % vitamin A as beta-carotene
- Vitamin C
- Calcium
- Iron
- Other added nutrients

Figure12-1 provides an example of a typical food label.

Serving sizes, listed at the top under the title, have long been an issue with nutritionists when a package that appears to be one serving may actually be two or two and a half, as with a 20-oz soda. When you eat a whole box of macaroni and cheese or a can of soup, it may be two servings, yet the information on the label is for one serving. That means all nutrient values should be multiplied by two.

The % Daily Value (DV) column helps you figure how much of a nutrient you are getting from a food that contributes to your total daily intake. If a label has 25% for vitamin A, it means you have to accumulate 75% from other food the rest of the day to reach 100% of the recommended intake. Sodium, saturated fat, and sugars are the three listed nutrients you want to keep track of to make sure you are not getting more than you need. Excess of these three may lead to serious heart problems, hypertension, and obesity.

Calories per serving appear on the label under serving size. It is important to know how many calories per day you eat to compute your DV of nutrients. Although the labels are based on a 2,000-calorie diet, as explained at the bottom in the footnote, it is recommended that women in the age group of 35 to 70 restrict their diet to 1,600 to 1,800 calories per day, and men in the same age group consume 2,000 to 2,200 calories per day.[1] Depending whether you are male or female and active or sedentary, you may have to increase or decrease the rest of the day's nutrients. Computing the DV for nutrients would then require a good pair of reading glasses and a calculator.

Ingredients

Ingredients are listed from the most abundant ingredient to the least abundant. For example, on a loaf of bread, you would assume the first ingredient listed would be bread flour, or beans on a can of green beans. Two facts are very important to remember when looking at this section, because there are two ingredients that may appear to be "hidden":

1. Sugars are sometimes listed separately, but if added together would be the first ingredient. Box 12-1 lists names of sugar.

2. Anything partially hydrogenated affects the body the same way as saturated fat. Box 12-2 lists examples of trans fats.

Label for Condensed
Tomato Soup

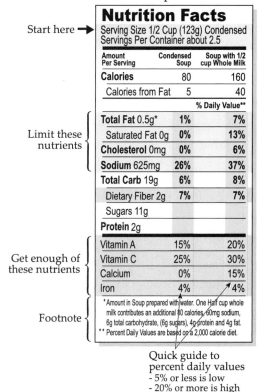

Figure 12-1. Nutrition label for condensed tomato soup.

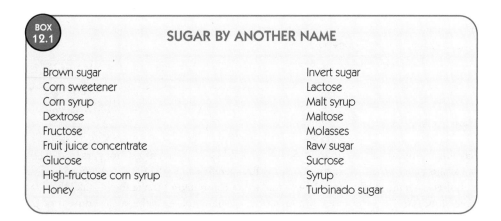

BOX 12.2

TRANS FATS

Partially hydrogenated corn oil
Partially hydrogenated soybean oil
Partially hydrogenated cottonseed oil
Fully hydrogenated vegetable oil

Table 12-1. FDA Requirements to Meet Health Claims

Health Claim	Requirements to Meet
Fat-free	1/2 g of fat/serving or less
Low-fat	3 g of fat/serving or less
Less fat	25% less fat than original recipe
Light (fat)	50% less fat than original recipe
Saturated fat-free	1/2 g of saturated or trans fat/serving or less
Cholesterol-free	2 g or less saturated fat/serving and less than 2 mg cholesterol/serving
Low cholesterol	2 g or less saturated fat/serving and less than 20 mg cholesterol/serving
Reduced calorie	25% fewer calories than original recipe
Low calorie	40 calories or less/serving
Light (calories)	1/3 fewer calories than original recipe
Extra lean	5 g fat or less, 2 g saturated fat or less, 95 mg cholesterol/100 g serving of meat, poultry, or seafood
Lean	10 g fat or less, 4 1/2 g saturated fat or less, 95 mg cholesterol/100 g serving of meat, poultry, or seafood
High fiber	5 g or more/serving
Sugar-free	1/2 g or less/serving
Sodium-free (salt-free)	1/2 g or less/serving
Low sodium	140 mg or less per serving
Very low sodium	35 mg or less/serving

Health Claims

Health claims are posted on the front of the food package to entice shoppers looking for a certain benefit from their food. The NLEA specifies which claims are allowed and the requirements the food has to meet to make that claim. Don't make the mistake that "fat-free" foods are "calorie-free." Manufacturers usually increase the sugar content of fat-

---

Table 12-2. Meanings of Health Claims

Health Claim	Meaning
Healthy	Low in fat, saturated fat, cholesterol, and sodium and has at least 10% DV of protein, iron, calcium, fiber, and vitamins A and C
Good source of, more, added	10% more DV of given nutrient than original recipe
High, rich in, excellent source of	20% or more of the given nutrient/serving
Less, fewer, reduced	25% less of given nutrient than original recipe
Low, little, few, low source of	Frequent consumption of food will not exceed DV

---

free foods to make up for what is lost by reducing the fat content. The texture of fat is lost but the taste is not compromised. Table 12-1 explains the FDA requirements that must be met to make certain health claims, and Table 12-2 explains the meaning of certain health claims.

Box 12-3 lists words that are not FDA approved as health claims.

Common Mistakes When Reading Labels

There are five common mistakes made when reading labels.

1. Forgetting that all label values are based on a 2,000-calorie diet. If you eat fewer or more than 2,000 calories, an adjustment must be made.

2. Thinking "reduced-fat" or "reduced sodium" on the label means the food is low-fat or low-sodium. All it means is that the food has 25% less fat or sodium. If the amount of either was high to begin with, reducing by 25% won't make much of a difference.

3. Thinking the percent of DV is the percent of calories. If the DV is 20%, it means you have consumed 20% of the recommended nutrient for the day.

4. Assuming the amount of sugar on a label is all added sugar. If one of the ingredients naturally has sugar, such as an orange, the amount of sugar includes what the ingredient naturally brings to the product.

5. Not reading serving sizes. A can of soup is usually two or two and a half servings, so all values must be multiplied accordingly.

BOX 12.3   The words right, smart, and natural are not FDA approved as health claims.

Doing the Calculations

There are many reasons for reading a label other than to know what ingredients the product contains or whether it is "rich" in certain nutrients. For some people, it is most important to calculate how much fat or carbohydrates a product has. The word *kilocalorie*, shortened to kcal, is the correct way to refer to the energy produced by food and expended by our bodies, although it is more commonly referred to as *calorie*. Most food has a calorie value, or the ability to provide energy. Knowing how many calories per gram a nutrient provides is the first step in doing the calculations. The following are calorie values of three major nutrients plus alcohol:

- Carbohydrates: 4 calories/g
- Protein: 4 calories/g
- Fat: 9 calories/g
- Alcohol: 7 calories/g

Box 12-4 is a chart of nutrient calorie values.

When working with numbers, you have to use similar values to multiply or divide. That means that to find percentage of calories, both numbers have to be calories. One can't be grams and the other calories.

To compute the number of calories from grams:

1. Find the number of grams of the nutrient.

2. Multiply by 4 for carbohydrate or protein, or 9 for fat.

3. Your answer is the number of calories generated from the nutrient.

Example:

If there are 32 g of carbohydrate: 4×32 g = 128 calories.

If there are 14 g of fat: 9×14 g = 126 calories.

Fat is the primary nutrient that is restricted in daily diets, and the one that is usually factored from a label to determine if the food product is a healthy choice. To keep track of how much fat you have in your diet, computing the percent of calories that

BOX 12.4   **COMPUTING THE NUMBER OF CALORIES FROM GRAMS**

CHO 4 cal/g
PRO 4 cal/g
FAT 9 cal/g
ALCOHOL 7 cal/g

come from fat in a food will help you decide if it is something you want to include in your meal.

1. Find the total number of calories for a serving size.

2. Find the total number of calories from fat.

3. Divide the calories from fat by the total calories and multiply by 100 to get a percentage.

4. If it is more than 30%, it is probably not a good choice.

Counseling Patients

Reading labels is a learned skill. Teaching your patient how to read labels and how the information can work to improve their food choices can have a great impact on long-term health. The following are some suggestions when teaching your patients this important tool for food selection:

1. Suggest they bring in labels from:
   a. packages of their favorite foods
   b. packages of similar foods for comparison

2. Calculate a healthy range for calories consumed daily, taking into consideration their:
   a. age
   b. body size
   c. desired weight
   d. activity level

3. Identify the parts of the label for them:
   a. Serving size: point out that some containers have more than one serving size
   b. Total calories per serving and those from fat
   c. DV of nutrient values
   d. Ingredients: instruct about
      i. Hidden sugars
      ii. Trans fats
   e. Footnote: values are based on a 2,000-calorie diet

4. Explain the meaning of certain health claims.

5. Identify which nutrients are most important to your patient and explain how to obtain the percentage contained in a serving size.

6. Review common mistakes when reading labels.

PUTTING THIS INTO PRACTICE

1. If one serving of baked beans has 260 calories and the label says there are 2 g of fat per serving, how many calories are from fat?

2. If one serving of Toaster Strudel has 350 calories and 140 of those calories are from fat, what percent of the Toaster Strudel is fat?

3. If one cup of Cranapple juice has 160 calories with 30 g of carbohydrates, what percent of the calories are carbohydrates?

4. There are 1.5 g of protein in one serving of Campbell's Beef and Potato Soup. The can has two servings but you eat the whole can. How many grams of protein have you consumed?

5. If one serving of turkey breast has 60 calories and the label says that there are 1.5 g of fat per serving, how many calories are from fat?

6. If one serving of turkey breast has 60 calories with 13.5 of those calories being fat, what percent of the turkey breast is fat?

7. If one cup of Instant Breakfast has 250 calories with 30 g being carbohydrates, what percent of the Instant Breakfast is carbohydrate?

8. Compare labels for Campbell's and Healthy Choice chicken noodle soup. Which contains the most sodium per serving?

9. If a label states the DV for vitamin A is 25%, how much of the vitamin do you need to consume in other foods throughout the day? (See RDA in Chapter 5.)

CHAPTER QUIZ

1. Restaurants are required by law to provide consumers with nutrient content of foods they serve.
   a. True
   b. False

2. If a food package states "sugar-free" or "fat-free," it must not contain any sugar or fat.
   a. True
   b. False

3. If the wrapper on a loaf of bread claims it is reduced calorie, the bread has half as many calories as a regular loaf of bread.
   a. True
   b. False

4. How many calories are there in 2 g of fat?
   a. 18
   b. 8
   c. 10
   d. 2

5. Which of the following is another name for sugar as an ingredient?
   a. Tumeric
   b. Potato starch
   c. Powdered cellulose
   d. Lactose
   e. Citric powder

6. The label on Honey Nut Cheerios states that there is 25% DV of iron in one cup of cereal. How many cups of this cereal would give you 100% of the DV for iron?
   a. 2
   b. 3
   c. 4
   d. 5

7. A high-fiber nutrition claim means there are at least _____g of fiber per serving.
   a. 2.5
   b. 5
   c. 10
   d. 25

Web Resources

FDA Weighs Food Label Changes http://www.msnbc.com/news/996445.asp

National Heart, Lung, and Blood Institute—Tipsheet: Reading Food Labels http://nhlbisupport.com/chd1/Tipsheets/reading-labels-tips.htm

Quaker Oatmeal—What to Look for When Reading Food Labels http://www.quakeroatmeal.com/Wellness/Articles/HE_FoodLabels.cfm

Understanding What Food Labels Mean http://www.dummies.com/WileyCDA/DummiesArticle/id-386.html

U.S. Department of Agriculture—Guidance on How to Understand and Use the Nutrition Facts Panel on Food Labels http://vm.cfsan.fda.gov/~dms/foodlab.html

U.S. Food and Drug Adminstration—The Food Label http://www.fda.gov/opacom/backgrounders/foodlabel/newlabel.html

References

1. Burros M. US diet proposals reflect nation's lack of fitness. New York Times, September 10, 2003.

Suggested Readings

Department of Health and Human Services, Food and Drug Administration. Food labeling: trans fatty acids in nutrition labeling, nutrient content claims, and health claims. Final rule. Fed Regist. 2003;68(133):41433–41506

U.S. Department of Agriculture. Nutrition and your health: dietary guidelines for Americans. 5th Ed. Washington, D.C., 2000.

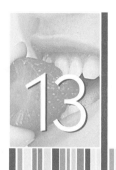

NUTRIENT NEEDS FOR DEVELOPMENT, GROWTH, AND MAINTENANCE OF ORAL STRUCTURES

Introduction

A well-educated, well-informed dental clinician can determine by a quick glance around the oral cavity whether a patient has been well-nourished during three phases of life: fetal development, preeruption of permanent teeth, and posteruption of permanent teeth. The oral cavity is a treasure chest of information regarding past and present nutritional choices and habits. Table 13-1 provides a list of nutrients and their effects and functions.

Effects of Diet During the Critical Period of Development

The critical period of development is the time during which the environment has the greatest impact on the developing embryo. The presence or absence of specific nutrients during fetal development can make the difference between health and disease of soft and hard structures. Mineralization of primary teeth begins during the third or fourth month of pregnancy. At birth, crowns of primary teeth are almost completely formed, and by the age of 1 year, calcification of the crowns of permanent teeth is mostly completed. Well-formed, well-calcified tooth structure can reduce the incidences of dental caries later in the life cycle. Presence or lack of other nutrients can make the difference between high-functioning salivary glands or those that are atrophied and produce little saliva. It also can make the difference between periodontal tissues that are resistant to bacterial invasion or those that have a tendency to pocket formation. Maternal nutrition plays a critical role in the fetus developing healthy oral structures. Although we have no control over the nutrition habits of our biological mothers, we can learn to develop healthy nutritional habits to countereffect any deficiencies that resulted in poorly formed hard and soft structures.

Table 13-1. Nutrients and Their Effects and Functions

Nutrient	Structure Affected	Other Function
Fat-Soluble Vitamins		
Vitamin A	Salivary glands Sulcular epithelium	
Vitamin D	Teeth—enamel, cementum Bone	Calcification of all hard tissues
Vitamin K		Blood clotting
Water-Soluble Vitamins		
Vitamin C	Collagen—dentin, pulp, cementum, alveolar bone, periodontal fibers, blood vessels, periodontal ligament	Wound healing
B-complex Cobalamine	Tongue, soft tissues	
Folacin		Deficiency may cause cleft lip and palate
Minerals		
Calcium	Enamel, cementum, bone	Calcification of all hard tissues
Phosphorus	Enamel, cementum, bone	Calcification of all hard tissues
Iron		Synthesis of hemoglobin
Zinc		Wound healing
Major Nutrients		
Protein	Maxilla, mandible, periodontal tissues	Repair and maintenance of tissues

Vitamin A

The general function of vitamin A is for synthesis of epithelial tissues.

- Preeruptively, vitamin A assists in the formation of mucous-secreting cells of the salivary glands and helps with the normal formation of enamel and dentin.
- Posteruptively, vitamin A maintains epithelial tissues and keeps the salivary glands working. It also maintains the integrity of the sulcular epithelium.

If there is a deficiency of vitamin A in the diet:

- Preeruptively, it could cause abnormal formation of enamel and dentin and contribute to the formation of cleft lip and/or palate and abnormal formation of salivary glands.

- Posteruptively, it could cause salivary glands to atrophy, reducing the amount of saliva available to the oral cavity. It could also hyperkeratinize normally thin, mucous membranes. Periodontal tissues can appear hyperkeratinized or hyperplastic with a tendency to pocket formation.

Vitamin D

The general function of vitamin D is to enhance absorption of calcium and phosphorous.

- Preeruptively, it aids with the calcification of all hard tissues—bone, enamel, dentin, and cementum.

- Posteruptively, it helps repair diseased bone.

If there is a deficiency of vitamin D in the diet:

- Preeruptively, it could cause enamel or dentin hypoplasia.

- Posteruptively, it could cause osteomalacia in adults and loss of lamina dura, as seen on dental radiographs. A deficiency results in an overall lack of mineralization of bone and cementum.

Vitamin K

Vitamin K aids with blood clotting time, so a deficiency of this nutrient could cause prolonged clotting time.

Vitamin C

Vitamin C helps with formation of collagen, which includes dentin, pulp, cementum, alveolar bone, periodontal fibers, blood vessels, gingival nerves, and periodontal ligament.

- Preeruptively, it helps with formation of bone and teeth and formation of all connective tissues.

- Posteruptively, it helps with formation of collagen, wound healing, and formation of connective tissues. It maintains the integrity of blood vessels and assists with phagocytosis.

A long-term deficiency in vitamin C results in the deficiency disease of scurvy. Oral appearance of scurvy mocks advanced, acute periodontal disease. Gingival tissues appear dark red to purple, spongy, and hemorrhagic, teeth are mobile, and breath is fetid. Its diagnosis is unusual in developed countries, but it is seen on rare occasions. If there is a mild deficiency of vitamin C:

- Preeruptively, it can cause irregular formation or absence of dentin.

- Posteruptively, it can cause enlarged, bluish-red, hemorrhagic gingival tissues.

B-Complex Vitamins

The B-complex vitamins are coenzymes and work together to maintain healthy oral tissues. Deficiencies can be seen in the oral cavity:

- Deficiency of thiamin (B-1) can cause the deficiency disease of beriberi. There is an increase in the sensitivity of oral tissues. The tongue burns and there is a general loss of taste.
- Deficiency of niacin (B-3) can cause the deficiency disease of pellagra. It affects the tongue, causing it to be sore, red, and swollen. Pain with eating and swallowing accompanies the symptoms.
- Deficiency of riboflavin (B-2) also affects the tongue, causing it to be inflamed. It also causes angular chelosis, and a greasy, red, scaly lesion resembling a butterfly shape can develop around the nose.
- Deficiency of cobalamine (B-12) causes pernicious anemia and a bright red, smooth, burning tongue.
- Deficiency of folacin also causes a burning tongue and oral mucosa, angular chelosis, gingivitis, and frequent oral lesions. There has been much research about the relationship between lack of folic acid during fetal development and cleft lips and palates.

Calcium and Phosphorus

Calcium and phosphorus are needed in abundance for calcification of hard tissues and need vitamin D to help with absorption.

- Preeruptively, they are responsible for mineralization of enamel, cementum, and bone.
- Posteruptively, they remineralize hard tissues and maintain bone.

If there is a deficiency of calcium and phosphorus in the diet:

- Preeruptively, it could cause hypocalcification of enamel.
- Posteruptively, it could allow bone loss.

Iron

Iron is needed for the synthesis of hemoglobin. A deficiency in the diet can cause glossitis and dysphagia (difficulty swallowing). The tongue's papilla atrophy and give a shiny, smooth, red appearance. It causes mucous membranes to appear ashen gray, as with anemia; it also can cause the occurrence of angular chelitis.

Zinc

Zinc is a mineral that helps with wound healing. A deficiency would cause a delay in wound healing and the epithelium of the tongue to thicken, which would decrease the sensation of taste.

Protein

Protein is known as the nutrient of repair and maintenance. It generally functions to help with formation and repair of all tissues.

- Preeruptively, it assists with the formation of maxilla, mandible, and periodontal tissues, and forms the matrix for enamel and dentin.
- Posteruptively, it repairs all tissues and forms antibodies to help resist infection

If there is a deficiency of protein in the diet:

- Preeruptively, it can slow the development of bone and tooth structure, which results in crowded and rotated teeth posteruptively. Crowded and rotated teeth lend themselves to increased caries susceptibility.
- Posteruptively, it can slow tissue healing and cause degeneration of periodontal connective tissues, including the periodontal ligament, bone, and cementum.

PUTTING THIS INTO PRACTICE

The last patient of the morning, a 35-year-old female, is new to your practice and presents for initial assessment. Her last dental visit was 6 years ago and she had a "deep cleaning" and a few fillings replaced at that time. Her chief complaint today is sore, bleeding gums.

Medical history is unremarkable.

Extra oral exam reveals:
- angular chelitis
- few facial moles
- infected bilateral ear piercing
- wearing of contacts

Intra oral exam reveals:
- Smooth, red tongue
- Amalgam tattoo buccal of #19
- Aphthous ulcer on labial near #25

Gingival exam reveals:
- Generalized marginal redness
- Heavy bleeding upon probing

Dental exam reveals:
- Past and present dental caries
- Impacted third molars
- Maxillary and mandibular anterior crowding

1. Based on the initial assessment information, comment on probable:
   a. Maternal nutrition during fetal development
   b. Preeruptive nutrition
   c. Posteruptive nutrition

CHAPTER QUIZ

1. The nutrient responsible for formation and proper functioning of saliva glands is:
   a. Vitamin D
   b. Iron
   c. Vitamin A
   d. Protein

2. The nutrient that aids absorption of calcium and phosphorus is:
   a. Vitamin K
   b. Vitamin A
   c. Vitamin D
   d. Folic acid

3. Two principle minerals that make up human enamel and are found under normal conditions in saliva are:
   a. Iron and calcium
   b. Calcium and magnesium
   c. Phosphorus and magnesium
   d. Calcium and phosphorus

4. Nutrients that have an effect on wound healing are:
   a. Vitamin C and zinc
   b. Vitamin D and calcium
   c. Vitamin A and B-complex
   d. Iron and zinc

5. A deficiency of which of the following nutrients can cause cleft palate?
   a. Protein
   b. Vitamin A
   c. Calcium
   d. Folic acid

6. Which of the following nutrients makes antibodies to resist infection?
   a. Vitamin A
   b. Protein
   c. Vitamin K
   d. Iron

7. Poor prenatal nutrition can cause an increase in caries risk later in life.

   a. True

   b. False

8. Lack of protein in a mother's diet during fetal development can cause a need for orthodontic intervention later in the child's life.

   a. True

   b. False

9. A deficiency of vitamin A in an adult's diet can cause hyperkeratosis of the gingival tissues and a tendency for periodontal pocket formation.

   a. True

   b. False

10. If you noticed loss of lamina dura on dental radiographs, you would suspect lack of which nutrient?

    a. Calcium

    b. Vitamin D

    c. Phosphorus

    d. Protein

    e. a, b, and c

Web Resources

American Dental Association—Tooth Eruption Charts www.ada.org/public/topics/tooth_eruption.asp

Cleft Palate Foundation—About Cleft Lip and Palate http://www.cleftline.org/aboutclp/

National Institute of Nutrition—The Effect of Diet on Dental Health http://www.nin.ca/public_html/Publications/NinReview/winter97.html

PBS—Folic Acid and Spina Bifida http://www.pbs.org/newshour/health/folic_acid/

Wide Smiles—Cleft Lip and Palate Resource http://www.widesmiles.org/

Suggested Readings

Alvarez JO, Caceda J, Woolley TW, Carley KW, Baiocchi N, Caravedo L, Navia JM. A longitudinal study of dental caries in the primary teeth of children who suffered from infant malnutrition. J Dent Res. 1993;72(12):1573–1576.

Alvarez JO. Nutrition, tooth development, and dental caries. J Coll Surg Edinb. 2001;46(6):320–328.

DePaola DP, Kuftinec MM. Nutrition in growth and development of oral tissues. Am J Clin Nutr. 1995;61(2):410S–416S.

Dreizen S. The mouth as indicator of internal nutritional problems. Int J Vitam Nutr Res. 1979;49(2):220–228.

Dreizen S. Nutrition and the immune response—a review. Int J Vitam Nutr Res 1979;49(2):220–228.

Palmer CA. Diet and Nutrition in Oral Health. Upper Saddle River, NJ: Prentice Hall, 2003.

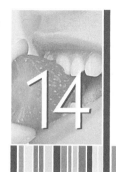

14

DIETARY CONSIDERATIONS FOR THE LIFECYCLE

Introduction

Good nutrition is vital for growth and health on the life continuum. Eating well is important before a mother becomes pregnant and continues to be important until death. Our bodies require the same basic nutrients our entire lives, but the recommended *quantities* for each vary as our physiologic needs change with aging.

General information on what to include in our diets to keep our bodies healthy for each stage of the lifecycle can be found in basic nutrition textbooks. Included in this chapter are highlights of those recommendations and how the diet relates to the oral cavity at a specific point in the growth continuum. Box 14-1 lists stages of the lifecycle.

Oral Health Throughout the Lifecycle

Prenatal

Ideally, a woman wishing to conceive should prepare her body by practicing good nutrition months before. Unfortunately, many women are unaware of their pregnancy in the early months, and by then, tooth development is already underway.

BOX 14.1	STAGES OF THE LIFECYCLE	
Prenatal–fetal		
Infant–birth:	12 months	
Toddler:	1–4 years	
Child:	5–12 years	
Teenager: 1	3–19 years	
Young Adult:	20–50 years	
Older Adult:	51 years and older	

If a mother is overweight or underweight throughout pregnancy, it increases her chance of complications. Aiming for optimal weight and health before conception, during pregnancy, and after delivery will give the child the greatest start in life.

- Obesity increases the mother's chance of developing life-threatening diseases for herself and her fetus. There is an increased incidence of hypertension, diabetes, preeclampsia, and prolonged delivery for the mother and congenital central nervous system malformations for the fetus.
- A pregnant mother who is severely underweight during pregnancy can be anemic and experience early delivery of a low–birth-weight baby.

There are three "myths" often heard about pregnancy that, in spite of a body of scientific study, have never been supported:

1. Eating for two
2. You lose a tooth for each child
3. Pregnant women crave unusual foods

Although the mother is eating to nourish herself and a baby, her body only requires an extra 300 calories per day beginning in the fourth month until delivery. The pregnant woman should try not to waste those 300 calories on simple carbohydrates and should consider including:

- extra protein for fetal tissue synthesis
- calcium for bone mineralization
- foods rich in all the B-complex vitamins for increase in energy metabolism
- fluids for the 25% increased need to support increase in maternal blood volume

A woman planning on becoming pregnant should make sure there are plenty of folate-rich foods in her diet or take a supplement containing at least 400 mcg of folic acid. Studies have shown that women with a folate deficiency during pregnancy have a greater chance of having a child with a neural tube defect. Box 14-2 provides a list of neural tube defects, and Box 14-3 provides a list of foods rich in folate.

Many people still believe that a mother can lose "one tooth per child" because the growing baby draws calcium from the mother's teeth. There has been no evidence to support this theory, although there is a correlation between motherhood and periodontal disease, due to stress.[1] If teeth are lost during pregnancy, it is usually due to decay and pain. If the mother has sufficient calcium in her diet, there will be enough calcium avail-

BOX 14.2

NEURAL TUBE DEFECTS

- Spina bifida: embryonic failure of fusion of one or more vertebral arches
- Malformation of the brain and skull
- Anencephaly: absence of bones of the cranial vault and cerebral and cerebellar hemispheres
- Encephalocele: gap in the skull with herniation of the brain

BOX 14.3

FOODS RICH IN FOLATE

Dark-green leafy vegetables
Citrus fruit and juices
Fortified cereal
Broccoli
Asparagus
Legumes
Beans
Peas
Nuts

able for the growing fetus. Early in the pregnancy, hormones cause an increase in calcium absorption and storage in the mother's body. If calcium is deficient in the diet, it may be taken from the mother's bones, where it has been stored for rapid fetal bone growth during the third trimester, but not from the teeth.

Pregnancy creates an altered sense of taste and smell. A pregnant woman may find she loses a taste for foods she once relished and that other foods smell bad and are no longer desired. Because of the changes in these two senses, eating patterns may seem very different. It is estimated that somewhere between 75% to 90% of women experience at least one food craving and 50% to 85% have at least one food aversion while pregnant. Most food cravings are for something sweet, such as ice cream. As with nonpregnant women, these cravings have been linked with emotional needs or changes in hormones. Box 14-4 lists food categories that are most often craved.

Some pregnant women report symptoms of pica—a condition where a person will crave and eat nonnutritive substances like dirt and laundry detergent. It is usually an indication of iron or other mineral deficiency but is not contingent on pregnancy.

Foods rich in calcium, phosphorus, and vitamin D are important in the pregnant woman's diet for healthy tooth formation. Tooth development begins as early as the sixth week after conception, and calcification of the primary teeth begins at 4 months in utero. Formation (not calcification) of many of the permanent teeth has already started by the time the baby is born. Table 14-1 charts tooth development for primary and permanent dentition.

Foods that can carry food-borne illnesses and should be avoided while pregnant are raw eggs, meat, soft cheeses, and unpasteurized juice. Some herbs can also be harmful to the fetus and should only be taken if prescribed by the doctor.

BOX 14.4

Sweets:	40%
Salty:	33%
Spicy:	17%
Sour:	10%

Table 14-1. Tooth Development

Tooth	Time of Formation
Primary incisors	4–5 mo in utero
Primary molars	5–6 mo in utero
Permanent central incisors	3–4 mo
Permanent lateral incisors	10–12 mo (3–4 mo mandible)
Permanent canine	4–5 mo
Permanent premolars	$1^{1}/_{2}$–$2^{1}/_{2}$ yr
Permanent first molars	At birth
Permanent second molars	$2^{1}/_{2}$–3 yr

Infant

Infancy is a time of tremendous growth—weight usually triples by the first birthday. Two facts about this time period: Intestinal absorption is inefficient and renal function is immature. With this in mind, infant nutrition must be specialized. Breast milk and infant formula both contain all the nutrients necessary for this time of rapid growth and should be provided exclusively for infants aged 4 to 6 months. Cow's milk has higher protein content than breast milk or formula and taxes the kidneys, so it is not recommended until after the age of 1. Introduction of solid foods should be handled one at a time so that possible allergies can be identified. By the age of 1 year, the infant's immature motor development allows the infant to attempt to feed him- or herself with a spoon or grab a cup, and the diet changes to include more variety.

Toddler

Toddlers are moving from a fluid diet to one that consists of more solid foods. This is the time for parents to set a good example, because eating habits learned as a toddler can last a lifetime. Toddlers can become "picky eaters." There is usually a decrease in appetite because rate of growth has dropped. Appetites will be erratic, but toddlers should not be forced to eat when they are not hungry. The National Health and Nutrition Examination Survey of 2000 reported that eating without hunger leads to overfeeding, which could possibly lead into childhood obesity. Fifteen percent of 6- to 19-year-olds are overweight. Box 14-5 lists pediatrician recommendations for total fat intake for toddlers.

It is not uncommon for toddlers to request the same foods for lunch and dinner in the same day, or for 5 days in a row. Because their calorie requirement has decreased, it

BOX 14.5

High cholesterol levels have been noted in children as young as 2 years old.

Pediatricians recommend that fat intake be kept around 30% of total daily calorie intake up to the age of 5 years.

BOX 14.6

HEALTHY SNACK SUGGESTIONS

- Sliced apples, pears, peaches, and grapes
- Slivers of carrots or celery with dip
- Bagels topped with peanut butter, smashed fruit, or cream cheese
- Soft taco rolls filled with leftover meat
- Cheese strips or cubes
- Yogurt
- Small crustless sandwiches
- Popcorn
- Peanut butter or cheese on crackers
- English muffin pizzas
- Tortillas with bean dip

is important for parents to guide their food choices to get the most nutrients from food. Snacking is an important part of the diet at this stage, so it is important to provide nutritious snack food versus snacks detrimental to teeth, such as fermentable carbohydrates.

Children have a tendency to model their eating patterns after parents. If fast food is a staple in the diet, now is the time to teach children to make healthier food choices. Thirty percent of all children report eating fast foods on any given day.[2] Milk or water instead of soda, and a salad instead of french fries will go a long way in fostering healthy eating habits in other lifecycle stages. Box 14-6 lists healthy snack choices for toddlers.

School-Age Child

The period when children are in school continues the time when they form a lifelong relationship with food. Although the brain is the same size as the adult's, the liver—where glucose is stored—is only about half as big. To maintain a steady blood glucose level, children need to eat more frequently—about every 4 hours. When children are not able to eat, their brains are depleted of glucose, which makes it difficult to concentrate in school.

Food takes on social, emotional, and psychological implications. Preference for comfort foods can last a lifetime, and other food choices may take on reward significance. Rewarding a child with sweets can be a hard habit to break later in life. Box 14-7 asks questions that help determine food's social, emotional, and psychological implications.

The school-age child's appetite is usually very good, with snacks making up the majority of the daily calories. Snacks provide the child with calories needed to maintain high energy levels. At this stage, children enjoy most foods, but as one can imagine, vegetables are last choice. Children can be ravenous after school and head toward the refrigerator as soon as they return home. Stocking up on ready-to-eat healthy snacks can be a quick fix for their hunger. Many snacks are bought from fast food restaurants and vending machines, but these food choices are high in fat, sugar, and salt and low in fiber. If the majority of daily calories are from these snacks, children's bodies will become deficient in major nutrients. Studies show that the low-nutrient food selections at fast food

BOX
14.7

SOCIAL, EMOTIONAL, AND PSYCHOLOGICAL IMPLICATIONS OF FOOD

- When you think of being sick, do you think of a specific food?
- When you feel happy and successful, do you reach for a certain food?
- What foods remind you of being with friends?
- What is your all-time favorite food?
- When you feel sad, do you reach for a particular food?

restaurants and vending machines contribute to the number of overweight children.[3] Parents should discourage day-long grazing and beverage sipping and set regular times for family meals to reduce both the caries potential of the diet and excess caloric intake. Vitamin/mineral supplements are very important as a back-up to an inadequate diet.

An increase in calcium is needed at this age. There is exfoliation of primary teeth, eruption of permanent teeth, and a growth spurt in long bones. A diet rich in calcium, phosphorus, and vitamin D should be continued for healthy development of bones and teeth.

Females begin to require more iron as menstruation begins. This is also a time when they become aware of their body image. Parents should use caution with their own projection of body image, because this can influence how a growing young woman feels about her own body.

Teenagers

Teenagers have the worst diets of any age group. Their diets are influenced by everyone and everything, except their parents: peer pressure, acne control, weight control, and muscle building. The teenage years are a period of very rapid physical growth, second only to infancy, and of intense stress and change. Hormonal changes affect every body organ, including the brain. About half of adult bone structure is deposited during adolescence and continues another 10 years. Nutrient and energy needs are greatly accelerated.

More responsibility is added to teenagers' lives as they obtain driver's licenses, begin dating, and work part-time jobs. Their busy lifestyles can dictate when, where, and what they eat. Unfortunately, their food selection usually does not meet their increased energy needs. Teenagers' favorite foods have been identified as hamburgers, pizza, fried chicken, Tex-Mex, french fries, spaghetti, ice cream, orange juice, and soda. Sodas replace milk and fruit juice, which causes inadequate calcium intake. Teenagers drink twice as much soda as milk, whereas the opposite was true 20 years ago. The average male drinks two cans per day and the female slightly less. That amounts to over 868 cans of soda per teenager each year, with a price tag of $54 billion yearly.

This is also an age when nutrient requirements differ for males and females. Females have reached their maximum linear growth and begin to increase their percentage of body fat. Males, on the other hand, are building up to their maximum linear growth and begin to develop more bone and muscle mass. A 15-year-old male can consume 4,000 calories per day just to maintain his current weight. More calories should be added for the extra energy needs. Table 14-2 compares the difference in growth and nutrient needs between males and females.

Both genders place tremendous importance on body shape and image during the teenage years. Females may worry they are not thin enough and males may worry they are not as muscular as they should be. The roots of many eating disorders begin at this stage, and if allowed to progress can be a lifelong battle to remain mentally and physically healthy. Considerations for teenage diet influence:

- Rate of very rapid growth
- Eat a typically unhealthy diet
- Nutrient needs for males and females differ
  - Females need more calcium and iron
  - Males have an increase in all major nutrient needs
- Food choices are influenced by peers
- Heightened awareness of body shape

Adulthood

Twenty-first century adults are very busy people. Lunch is usually eaten away from home, many meals are skipped, and dinner is prepared as quickly as possible. It is a time of multiple stresses and multitasking: raising children, managing a home, and keeping track of both household and work schedules. In spite of all this "busyness," nutrient needs are reduced. There is a gradual slowing of metabolic rate that goes unnoticed at first, but emerges to consciousness somewhere around the age of 50. Adults will notice that they may eat less and still gain weight. Organ function begins to become less efficient around the age of 30 and continues to decline as we age. Just as you notice subtle changes in texture, color, and amount of hair as well as a "loosening" of the skin, internal organs are also going through gentle changes in function. All senses begin to diminish. Ability to see and hear slowly fades and can make reading labels and recipes difficult.

Table 14-2. Growth and Nutrient Needs for Males and Females

Males	Females
Maximum linear growth is hit at 15	Maximum linear growth is hit at 13
Eat twice as much as females of same age	Interested in achieving a slender figure through calorie reduction
2,500 cal for ages 11–14 3,000 cal for ages 15–18	2,200 cal for ages 11–18
	Need more iron because of monthly blood loss

Inability to taste well may lead to overseasoning. The thirst mechanism begins to fail, which can cause dehydration. Consideration for adult diet influence:

- Metabolic rate slows.
- Organ function begins to diminish.
- Sight and hearing are impaired.
- Taste sensation is reduced.
- There is an inability to sense thirst.
- There is an overall reduced enjoyment of food.

Elderly

With the state of our current medical technology, life expectancy has increased and some people live into their 100s. Studies are ongoing about the calorie-reduction diet and its relationship to longevity. The elderly age group is different from those previously mentioned in that biologic age varies widely with chronological age. A person who has reached the age of 70 could have a biologic age of a 50-year-old, and vice versa. Depending on genetics, life experiences, and ability to resist disease, our bodies age at different rates. Good nutrition plays an important role in keeping the body free from disease and the dentition healthy. From the age of 50, calorie intake should decrease and physical activity should increase. Lean body mass declines (due to decrease in protein intake) and adipose tissue increases.

Many elderly patients will report taking multiple medications, most of which cause xerostomia. Eating with a very dry mouth becomes uncomfortable. Foods will stick to teeth and soft tissues, allowing spicy foods to burn unlubricated mucosa. Each bolus of food might seem to "stick" going down. This can lead to eliminating dry, sticky, and crunchy foods and adding soft, bland items to the diet. With a higher incidence of root caries and periodontal disease at this stage, good nutrition is very important to maintain a healthy dentition. Loss of teeth makes chewing difficult, and the elimination of crunchy foods with meals minimizes the flow of good saliva. Teeth don't get the good buffering effects of sodium bicarbonate, calcium, and phosphorus. The following list includes some common reasons for poor eating habits of the elderly:

- Dysphagia: swallowing problems
- Altered GI motility: constipation lining of intestinal tract is not replaced as often
- Economic: fixed incomes mean a greater percentage of the elderly at poverty level, with failing health and high medical bills
- Psychological: apathy and depression cause decreased appetite and interest in food
- Side effects of medication and social factors (inability to drive, living alone); most of their friends may have passed on
- Eating meals out frequently: meet in groups at fast food restaurants for socialization and to take advantage of senior discounts

Counseling Patients

Pregnancy

- Prenatal vitamins are a good idea, even if just considering a pregnancy.
- Don't eat twice as much just because you are "eating for two." Around the fourth month of pregnancy, increase daily calorie intake by 300 but include extra protein, calcium, and food rich in vitamins and minerals in those extra calories.
- Get at least 400 mcg of folate in your diet or supplement to prevent neural tube defects.
- Increase fluid intake.
- Avoid caffeine, alcohol, tobacco, and any drug not prescribed by your physician. All pass through the placental barrier and affect the growing child.
- Minimize processed foods from the diet because all have artificial colorants and flavoring, and it is not well-known how these affect the growing child.
- Take adequate iron to avoid iron-deficiency anemia.
- Adequate calcium, phosphorus, and vitamin D intake ensures good calcification of your child's teeth.

Infancy

- If formula is made with distilled or bottled water that does not contain fluoride, ask the pediatrician if fluoride supplementation is needed.
- Primary teeth are beginning to erupt into the oral cavity. Prevent early childhood caries by not putting the infant to bed with a bottle. Fluid pools around teeth, causing dental caries.
- Use water to quench thirst and juice occasionally because of acidic pH that contributes to early childhood caries.
- The crowns of permanent teeth are in a stage of calcification, so adequate calcium, phosphorus, and Vitamin D are required.

Toddlers

- Have suggestions for healthy snacks readily available when counseling.
- Consider level of income and availability of foods.

School-Age Child

- Avoid using food as punishment, reward, or consolation.
- There is a tendency for the school-age child to choose soda over milk, but this practice should be discouraged.
- Involve children in meal preparation; they're more apt to eat what they cook.

Teenagers

- Appeal to their body image, such as muscular development.
- Praise good food choices and ignore the others.
- Encourage healthy snacks—cooked meats, nuts, cheese, milk, fruit, peanut butter, and popcorn.
- This is the time when young women should begin acquiring a surplus of calcium in their bones.

Adult

- Between 30 and 40, resorption of existing bone begins to exceed formation of new bone, resulting in a net loss of bone.
- Bone growth and shaping of the growing skeleton cease at maturity, and remodeling takes over.
- Bone loss happens in both males and females, and once it begins, it continues throughout the rest of life.
- Osteoporosis is the result of excessive bone loss.

Elderly

- The greatest reduction in nutrient and energy needs is in the elderly years.
- Increase fiber intake.
- Decrease fat intake.
- Recommend a senior vitamin/mineral supplement.
- Ensure adequate calcium intake to avoid osteoporosis.
- Multiple medications can alter how the body absorbs vitamins and minerals.
- There is an increased need for exercise, which will resist bone resorption for prevention of osteoporosis.
- The elderly may restrict fluid intake due to incontinence or nocturia.

PUTTING THIS INTO PRACTICE

1. Obtain an informational brochure on the nutrient content of foods served at two of your favorite fast food restaurants.
   a. Compare the fat, cholesterol, carbohydrates, and sodium for your favorite selections at each restaurant.

	Name of Restaurant	
Nutrient	First Selection	Second Selection
Saturated fat		
Total fat		
Cholesterol		
Carbohydrate		
Sodium		

   b. Is one choice better than the other?
   c. How could you boost the nutrient content of your selection and at the same time reduce fat and sodium?
   d. What would you suggest to improve the selections of a client who frequents fast food restaurants?

2. If your client asked your opinion on what to provide as an after-school snack for their school-age child, what suggestions would you give them?

3. Give an example of a healthy snack for each of the following age groups:
   a. Toddler
   b. School-Age Child
   c. Teenager
   d. Adult
   e. Elderly

CHAPTER QUIZ

1. Which of the following nutrients, if deficient during pregnancy, can cause neural tube defects?

   a. Protein

   b. Calcium

   c. Folic acid

   d. Vitamin B-12

2. Which of the following is an example of a neural tube defect?

   a. Incomplete closure of spinal cord

   b. Undersized auricular structure

   c. Incomplete development of nerve synapses

   d. Inability to digest protein

3. Which age group requires a *reduction* in energy and nutrient needs?

   a. Infant

   b. Toddler

   c. Teenager

   d. Elderly

   e. b and d

   f. None of the above

4. Which age group does the parent have the least amount of influence on in food choices?

   a. Infancy

   b. Toddler

   c. School-Age Child

   d. Teenager

Web Resources

Academy of General Dentistry—Children's Nutrition: What Foods Cause Tooth Decay in Children? http://www.agd.org/consumer/topics/childrensnutrition/main.html

Academy of General Dentistry—Development Chart for Feeding Infants http://www.agd.org/consumer/topics/childrensnutrition/weaningchart.html

American Dental Association—Good Oral Health Begins in the Womb http://www.ada.org/public/media/releases/0202_release06.asp

Better Food Choices at Fast Food Restaurants (from the Minnesota Attorney General) http://www.olen.com/food/book.html

Calorie Content of Fast Food http://www.diet-i.com/calorie_chart/fast-food.htm

Economic Research Service—Nutrient-to-Calorie Density http://www.ers.usda.gov/briefing/DietAndHealth/data/nutrients/table8.htm

Fast Food Finder by Olen Publishing http://www.olen.com/food/index.html

Fast Food Nutrition Fact Explorer http://www.fatcalories.com/

Ingredient List and Nutritional Counts of Select Restaurants http://www.dietriot.com/fff/rest.html

Living Longer: A History of Longevity http://www.pbs.org/stealingtime/living/history.htm

References

1. Scheutz F, Baelum V, Matee MI, Mwangosi I. Motherhood and dental disease. Community Dent Health 2002;19(2):67–72.

2. Bowman SA, Gortmaker SL, Ebbeling CB, Pereira MA, Ludwig DS. Effects of fast-food consumption on energy intake and diet quality among children in a national household survey. Pediatrics 2004;113(1):112–118.

3. Hurley J, Liebman B. Kid's cuisine, what would you like with your fries? Nutrition Action Healthletter March 2004:12–15.

Suggested Readings

Berkey CS, Rockett HR, Gillman MW, Field AE, Colditz GA. Longitudinal study of skipping breakfast and weight change in adolescents. Int J Obes Relat Metab Disord. 2003;27(10):1258–1266.

Budtz-Jorgensen E, Chung JP, Rapin CH. Nutrition and oral health. Best Pract Res Clin Gastroenterol. 2001;15(6):885–896.

Chen C. Adolescent diets and oral health. Probe. 2004;38(1):16–20.

Collins K. Help for parents of picky eaters. MSNBC News, July 18, 2004.

Davis J, Stegeman C. The Dental Hygienists Guide to Nutritional Care. Philadelphia: W. B. Saunders, 1998.

Falco MA. The lifetime impact of sugar excess and nutrient depletion on oral health. Gen Dent. 2001;49(6):591–595.

Fitzsimons D, Dwyer JT, Palmer C, Boyd LD. Nutrition and oral health guidelines for pregnant women, infants, and children. J Am Diet Assoc. 1998;98(3):264.

French SA, Story M. Neumark-Sztainer D, Fulkerson JA, Hannan P. Fast food restaurant use among adolescents: associations with nutrient intake, food choices and behavioral and psychosocial variables. Int J Obes Relat Metab Disord. 2001;25(12):1823–1833.

Johnson SL. Improving preschoolers' self-regulation of energy intake. Pediatrics 2000;106(6):1429–1435.

Leung M, et al. Dietary intakes of preschoolers. J Am Diet Assoc 1984;84 (5):551–554.

Lucas A. Programming by early nutrition: an experimental approach. Presented as part of the symposium "The effects of childhood diet on adult health and disease" at the Experimental Biology 1997 meeting, New Orleans, 1997.

Marshall TA, Warren JJ, Hand JS, Xie XJ, Stumbo PJ. Oral health, nutrient intake and dietary quality in the very old. J Am Dent Assoc. 2002;133(10):1369–1379.

Mojon P, Budtz-Jorgensen E, Rapin CH. Relationship between oral health and nutrition in very old people. Age Ageing 1999;28(5):463–468.

Paeratakul S, Ferdinand DP, Champagne CM, Ryan DH, Bray GA. Fast-food consumption among US adults and children: dietary and nutrient intake profile. J Am Diet Assoc. 2003;103(19):1296–1297.

Palmer C. Diet and Nutrition in Oral Health. Upper Saddle River, NJ: Pearson Education, 2003.

Robin L. Healthy eating is essential for healthy teeth in young children. Probe. 2004;38(1):14–15.

Sahyoun NR, Lin CL, Krall E. Nutritional status of the older adult is associated with dentition status. J Am Diet Assoc. 2003;103(1):61–66.

Saunders MJ. Nutrition and oral health in the elderly. Dent Clin North Am. 1997;41(1):681–698.

Sheiham A, Steele J. Does the condition of the mouth and teeth affect the ability to eat certain foods, nutrient and dietary intake and nutritional status amongst older people? Public Health Nutr. 2001;4(3):797–803.

Sheiham A, Steele JG, Marcenes W, Tsakos G, Finch S, Walls AW. Prevalence of impacts of dental and oral disorders and their effects on eating among older people; a national survey in Great Britain. Community Dent Oral Epidemiol. 2001;29(3):195–203.

Utter J, Neumark-Sztainer D, Jeffery R, Story M. Couch potatoes or French fries: are sedentary behaviors associated with body mass index, physical activity, and dietary behaviors among adolescents? J Am Diet Assoc. 2003;103(10):1298–1305.

Vandewater EA, Shim MS, Caplovitz AG. Linking obesity and activity level with children's television and video game use. J Adolesc. 2004;27(1):71–85.

Vargas CM, Dye BA, Hayes KL. Oral health status of older rural adults in the United States. J Am Dent Assoc. 2003;134(4):479–486.

Walls AW, Steele JG, Sheiham A, Marcenes W, Moynihan PJ. Oral health and nutrition in older people. J Public Health Dent. 2000;60(4):304–307.

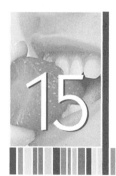

EATING DISORDERS

Introduction

Eating disorders are very private, secret, and personal, to the point where one who suffers may deny it publicly and refuse to seek treatment. Controlling food intake may be the only sense of control a person with an eating disorder may feel in their lives, and they won't give it up easily.

In the United States, 5 to 10 million females and 1 million males struggle with eating disorders. They affect mainly adolescent girls, but diagnoses are increasing in the male population and other age groups. Treatment includes medication and psychiatric and nutritional counseling. The earlier in the disease process treatment is begun, the more successful it is. Unfortunately, 5% to 20% of those affected by eating disorders will succumb to death.

Etiology is multifactorial and is influenced by social, psychological, biologic, and cultural factors. Each disorder may have distinct physical symptoms with oral manifestations, and it is the oral complications that eventually lead the patient with an eating disorder to the dental office. Since the dental auxiliary is the person most likely to take the medical/dental history and provide the first oral exam, he or she may also be the first to identify the disease. Dental auxiliaries usually are not regarded as people of authority or as threatening to the patient, and because of this, they are usually the perfect choice for a confidant. Counseling and treatment for the specific eating disorder is not among the dental professional's responsibilities, but restoring oral problems and prevention of oral complications caused by the disease are both necessary and expected.

There are three main eating disorders:

- Anorexia nervosa
- Bulimia nervosa
- Binge eating

BOX 15.1 — FACTORS INVOLVED IN EATING DISORDERS

- Psychological
- Social/Interpersonal
- Biologic

Etiology of Eating Disorders

Eating disorders are not something that one catches, but rather something that one develops. They stem from psychological, social/interpersonal, and biologic situations that lead to a preoccupation with food. Box 15-1 lists factors involved in eating disorders.

Psychological Factors:

- Low self-esteem
- Feelings of inadequacy or lack of control in life
- Depression, anxiety, anger, and loneliness

Social/Interpersonal Factors:

- Media pressure that misrepresents perfectly thin bodies as being preferable
- Nonacceptance of beauty in diversity (narrow views)
- Difficulty with family and interpersonal relationships
- Difficulty in expressing emotions and feelings
- History of being teased about weight
- History of sexual abuse

The media play a huge role in propagating eating disorders by employing unnaturally thin models and insinuating that all should aspire to look like them. The following are facts referenced on the National Eating Disorders Association's (NEDA) website:

- 80% of American women are dissatisfied with their appearance.
- The average American woman is 5'4" tall and weighs 140 pounds. Compare that to the average American model, who is 5'11" tall and weighs 117 pounds.
- Most fashion models are thinner than 98% of American women.
- 81% of 10-year-olds are afraid of being fat.
- 51% of 9- and 10-year-olds feel better about themselves if they are on a diet.
- 91% of women on college campuses attempt to control their weight through dieting.
- 95% of all dieters will regain their lost weight in 1 to 5 years.
- $40 billion is spent on dieting and diet-related products each year.

Biologic Factors

- Unbalanced brain chemicals that signal and control hunger and satiety

Anorexia Nervosa

Anorexia nervosa is mainly a disease witnessed in young females shortly after puberty or during adolescence. Its characteristic self-imposed weight loss regime stems from a distorted attitude toward eating and body weight. Anorexics appear painfully thin, and even though they look like skin on a skeleton, in their minds they still look fat. Food is the enemy, and every minute of every day the anorexic is thinking of ways to lose weight. This self-imposed starvation wreaks havoc on the body. If it is left untreated, an electrolyte imbalance can cause cardiac arrest and, ultimately, death.

Signs and Symptoms:

- Terrified of gaining weight
- Excuses for not eating meals
- Cook for others then don't eat themselves
- Excessive use of diuretics and laxatives
- Low self-esteem—may feel like they don't deserve to eat
- Excessive exercise
- Strive for perfection
- Put needs of others before their own
- Distorted self-image
- Self-worth is dependent on weight—they frequently check their weight
- Know more about caloric content of foods than specialists
- May wear baggy clothes to cover up thinness or inappropriate clothing for the season (wearing a coat in summer)

Physical Symptoms of Anorexia:

- Fatigue and muscle weakness
- Irregular or absence of menstruation (amenorrhea)
- Fainting or dizziness
- Pale complexion (pallor)
- Headaches
- Irregular heartbeats
- Cold hands and feet
- Loss of bone mass
- Electrolyte imbalance

- Insomnia
- Low potassium—cardiac arrest

Oral Signs of Anorexia:

- Anemic tissues
- Chapped lips

You may notice the following physical symptoms of a person with anorexia nervosa when the person is in your chair:

- Painfully thin
- May have appearance of lanugo—a light fuzzy hair on face
- Avoids eye contact
- Dehydration
- Dry brittle skin and nails
- Low blood pressure, lowered metabolic rate, and always cold

Bulimia Nervosa

Bulimics are of normal-looking weight. The classic symptom of this disease is binging on food and then purging. A diagnosis is made if binging/purging occurs at least twice a week for at least 3 months. It is a cycle of overeating, feeling guilty about overeating, purging, and then feeling relief. The amount of food used to binge can vary according to the perception of the person who suffers from this disorder. For some, eating one cookie may be binging, and for others, it may be eating two whole packages of cookies, a whole pizza, and a half-gallon of ice cream in one sitting. Purging can be by way of vomiting, use of laxatives and/or enemas, excessive exercising, fasting, and use of diuretics and/or diet pills. Vomiting with the help of the first two fingers down the throat is the most reported means of purging. Many times, a callous will develop on the fingers used to help purge because they rub against the central incisors. Figure 15-1 illustrates the cycle of binging and purging.

Signs and Symptoms of Bulimia:

- Binge eating
- Visits bathroom immediately after eating
- Vomiting
- Misuse of laxatives and diuretics
- Use of diet pills
- Fasting
- Depression
- Excessive exercising
- Avoids restaurants and planned social meals

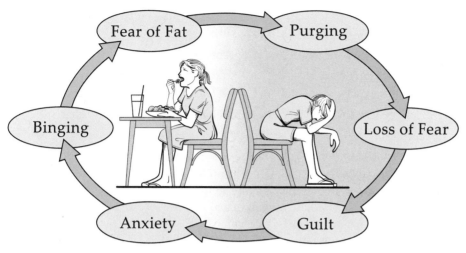

Figure 15-1. Binging and purging cycle.

Physical Signs of Bulimia:

- Broken blood vessels in eyes
- Fatigue
- Muscle weakness
- Irregular heartbeats
- Dizziness
- Headaches
- Dehydration
- Amenorrhea
- Electrolyte imbalance and low blood pressure
- Chest pains
- Stomach ulcers
- Edema in hands and feet
- Cardiac arrest
- Death

Gastric acids that pass through the oral cavity can leave clues for you, indicating your client is a bulimic.

Oral Signs of Bulimia:

- Enamel erosion/brittle enamel
- Dentinal hypersensitivity
- Extrusion of amalgam restorations

- Xerostomia
- Swollen parotid glands
- Erythematous oral tissues and red palate
- Chronic sore throat
- Chapped lips
- Moderate to severe dental caries (from binge-food selection)
- Pain
- Unaesthetic appearance of teeth

Many of the symptoms of anorexia and bulimia overlap, and it is not uncommon for an anorexic to also be bulimic. Table 15-1 compares symptoms of anorexia nervosa and bulimia nervosa. Figure 15-2 demonstrates the overlap in eating disorder symptoms. Figure 15-3 lists some of the symptoms of anorexia nervosa.

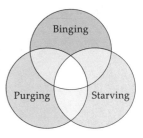

Figure 15-2. Overlap of eating disorders.

Binge Eating

There is no mistaking a binge eater. They eat a great amount of food in a short period of time, usually by themselves. They eat until they are uncomfortably full, many times when they are not even hungry, and end up feeling disgusted, depressed, and guilty for eating so much. The difference between the bulimic binging and the binge eater is that a binge eater does not purge, so all the calories end up making them obese. Obesity further complicates their life by adding risk for associated diseases.

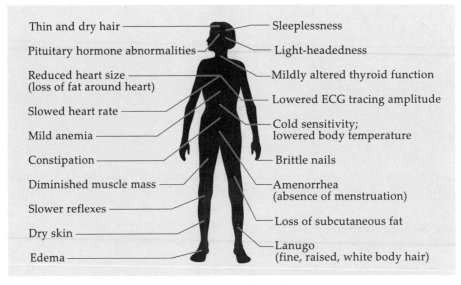

Figure 15-3. Symptoms of anorexia nervosa.

Table 15-1. Symptoms of Anorexia and Bulimia

Symptom	Anorexia	Bulimia
Weight loss	X	
Weight fluctuation		X
Secretive eating		X
Binge eating		X
Fasting	X	X
Food obsession	X	
Use of laxatives	X	X
Use of diuretics	X	X
Use of diet pills	X	X
Purging		X
Heavy exercising	X	X
Wear inappropriate clothing	X	
Uncomfortable around food	X	
Frequent checking of weight	X	
Psychological Depression	X	X
Low self-esteem	X	X
Withdrawn	X	
Guilt	X	X
Perfectionistic	X	
Physical Fatigue	X	X
Always cold	X	
Broken vessels		X
Swollen glands	X	X
Muscle weakness	X	X
Lanugo	X	
Amenorrhea	X	X
Menstrual irregularities	X	X
Dizziness	X	X
Fainting	X	
Dehydration	X	X
Pallor	X	
Headaches	X	X
Dry skin and brittle hair	X	
Shortness of breath	X	X
Irregular heartbeats	X	X
Constipation	X	X
Low blood pressure	X	X
High blood pressure		X
Electrolyte imbalance	X	X
Chest pains		X
Gastric problems		X
Edema	X	X
Loss of bone mass	X	
Insomnia	X	
Anemia	X	X
Low potassium	X	
Cardiac arrest	X	X
Abrasions on index and middle finger		X
Death	X	X

Physical Symptoms of Binge Eating:

- Obesity
- Diabetes
- High blood pressure
- High cholesterol
- Osteoarthritis
- Decreased mobility
- Shortness of breath
- Heart disease
- Liver and kidney problems
- Cardiac arrest
- Death

Treatment

Treatment for all eating disorders involves medical intervention, psychological help, and nutritional counseling. Box 15-2 lists treatment strategies.

The sooner an eating disorder is diagnosed, the better the outcome is. Antidepressants are usually prescribed once weight has been stabilized. Dental care is part of the recovery program. Oral effects of gastric acids and binging on cariogenic foods are usually the impetus for a visit to the dental office. Pain from erosion, dentinal sensitivity, and caries can get intense. Comprehensive dental treatment is usually postponed until behavior is changed so that tooth damage does not continue. Choice in restorative dental treatment depends on mental health status and the severity of damage to the teeth. Box 15-3 lists dental treatments provided.

- Composites, overlays, crowns, and veneers can restore the teeth, depending on the severity of erosion.
- Fluoride and sodium bicarbonate rinses can prevent further sensitivity and caries from acids and cariogenic foods.
- Restoring the teeth to a more aesthetic appearance helps increase self-esteem.

BOX 15.2 TREATMENT STRATEGIES FOR EATING DISORDERS

- Medical intervention
- Psychological counseling
- Nutritional counseling

BOX 15.3

DENTAL TREATMENT

Aesthetic Restorations
- Crowns
- Composites
- Veneers

Home Care Instructions
- Wait 30 minutes after purging before brushing.
- Rinse with sodium bicarbonate after purging.
- Use a fluoride mouthwash before retiring for the night.

Treatment for Sensitivity
- Use a toothpaste for sensitive teeth.
- Use a commercially available desensitizing agent such as Protect, Seal and Protect, Duraflor, Pain-Free, etc.

Lesser-Known Eating Disorders

- Compulsive overeating: uncontrollable eating and consequential weight gain. Food is used to comfort and destress. This is seen more frequently in males.

- Anorexia athletica: frantic exercising and fanatic about weight and diet. Time may be taken from school or work to exercise. People with this disease are rarely satisfied with physical achievements and move from one challenge to the next.

- Body dysmorphic disorder: excessively concerned about appearance and magnifies flaws. People with this body dysmorphic disorder may undergo multiple unneeded plastic surgeries.

- Orthorexia nervosa: excessive focus on eating pure or superior food. People with orthorexia nervosa usually obsess over what to eat and where to obtain it.

- Pica: craving and eating nonfood items like dirt, laundry detergent, cigarette butts, clay, chalk, paint chips, cornstarch, baking soda, coffee grounds, glue, toothpaste, and soap. Pica may accompany a developmental disorder such as autism, mental retardation, or brain injury.

Counseling Patients

The patient usually initiates a dental visit due to dental erosion, sensitivity, or aesthetic problems. The dental professional's role in treating patients with eating disorders is that of:

- case finder and referring to a medical professional
- restoring dental and oral tissues
- prevention

It is important to realize that a patient may relapse, so establishing regular recall visits to monitor dental care may prevent further damage.[1] When counseling patients with an eating disorder, take care in how your instructions are worded. Their self-esteem is usually very fragile and if they perceive the visit as not going well, they will not continue treatment. Avoid placing blame or shame, using accusatory statements, and giving simple solutions to their dental problems. Express continued support, even if they have a relapse. Home care instructions should include:

- Rinse with water and baking soda or magnesium hydroxide after vomiting.
- Use home fluoride rinses before retiring for the night.
- Don't brush for 30 minutes after purging—allow saliva to remineralize enamel.
- Limit intake of acidic beverages.
- Avoid sticky, sweet foods between meals.
- Suck on sugar-free chewing gum or sugar-free hard candies (lemon balls) to stimulate saliva.
- Educate about the oral effects of purging:
  - ditched amalgams
  - enamel erosion
  - sensitivity
  - irregular incisal edges
  - discolored teeth

PUTTING THIS INTO PRACTICE

1. Write out what you would say to a patient whom you suspect may be bulimic because of enamel erosion on the linguals of the maxillary anterior teeth and ditched amalgam fillings.
2. If the client admits to bulimic purging, what would you suggest as prevention for further oral problems?
3. Research local eating disorder clinics and treatment centers. Make a notecard of addresses and phone numbers for client referral to be accessed when needed.

CHAPTER QUIZ

1. Which eating disorder is characterized by binging and purging?
    a. Anorexia nervosa
    b. Bulimia nervosa
    c. Binge eating
    d. Anorexia athletica

2. Which eating disorder causes a person to crave nonfood items?
    a. Anorexia nervosa
    b. Body dysmorphic
    c. Pica
    d. Binge eating

3. Most American women are satisfied with their appearance.
    a. True
    b. False

4. Which eating disorder causes tooth sensitivity due to enamel erosion?
    a. Anorexia nervosa
    b. Pica
    c. Binge eating
    d. Bulimia nervosa
    e. Body dysmorphic

5. People with bulimia nervosa usually have high self-esteem because they are able to control their body weight.
    a. True
    b. False

6. Most binge eaters, once diagnosed and treated, are able to diet and obtain permanent weight loss.
    a. True
    b. False

7. It is not unusual for a person to be both anorexic and bulimic.
    a. True
    b. False

8. Clients should be instructed to brush immediately after vomiting to prevent gastric acids from eroding enamel.
    a. True
    b. False

Web Resources

Anorexia Nervosa and Related Eating Disorders http://www.anred.com/welcome.html

The National Eating Disorder Information Centre of Canada http://www.nedic.ca/

Academy for Eating Disorders http://www.aedweb.org/newwebsite/index.htm

Harvard Eating Disorders Center http://www.hedc.org/

National Eating Disorders Association http://www.nationaleatingdisorders.org/p.asp?WebPage_ID=337

The National Centre for Eating Disorders of the United Kingdom http://www.eating-disorders.org.uk/

Gurze Books—Eating Disorders Resources http://www.gurze.com/

Eating Disorder Referral and Information Center http://www.edreferral.com/

Overeaters Anonymous http://www.overeatersanonymous.org/

National Institute of Mental Health—Eating Disorders: Facts About Eating Disorders and the Search for Solutions http://www.nimh.nih.gov/publicat/eatingdisorders.cfm

National Women's Health Information Center—Body Image http://4women.gov/bodyimage/BodyImage.cfm?page=125

Body Positive—Boosting Body Image at Any Weight http://bodypositive.com

References

1. Studen-Pavlovich D, Elliott MA. Eating disorders in women's oral health. Dent Clin North Am. 2001;45(3):491–511.

Suggested Readings

Bonilla ED, Luna O. Oral rehabilitation of a bulimic patient; a case report. Quintessence Int. 2001;32(6):469–475.

Brown S, Bonifazi DZ. An overview of anorexia and bulimia nervosa, and the impact of eating disorders on the oral cavity. Compendium 1993;14(12):1594–1608.

Christensen GJ. Oral care for patients with bulimia. J Am Dent Assoc. 2002;133(12):1689–1691.

Diaz-Marsa M, Carrasco JL, Saiz J. A study of temperament and personality in anorexia and bulimia nervosa. J Personal disord. 2000;14(14):352–359.

Emans SJ. Eating disorders in adolescent girls. Pediatr Int. 2000;42(1):1–7.

Faine MP. Recognition and management of eating disorders in the dental office. Dent Clin North Am. 2003;47(2):395–410.

Goldie MP. Striving for thin. Dimensions of dental hygiene. 2004:32–33.

Gurenlian JR. Eating disorders. J Dent Hyg. 2002;76(3):219–234.

Hazelton LR, Faine MP. Diagnosis and dental management of eating disorder patients. Int J Prosthodont. 1996;9(1):65–73.

Howat PM, Varner LM, Wampold RL. The effectiveness of a dental/dietician team in the assessment of bulimic dental health. J Am Diet Assoc. 1990;90(8):1099–1102.

Little JW. Eating disorders: dental implications. Oral Surg Oral Med Oral Pathol Oral Radiol Endol. 2002;93(2):138–143.

Milosevic A. Eating disorders and the dentist. Br Dent J. 1999; 186(3):109–113.

Montecchi PP, Custureri V, Polimeni A, Cordaro M, Costa L, Marinucci S, Montecchi F. Oral manifestations in a group of young patients with anorexia nervosa. Eat Weight Disord. 2003;8(2): 164–167.

Muller JA. Eating disorders: identification and intervention. J Contemp Dent Pract. 2001;15(2):98.

Robb ND, Smith BG. Anorexia and bulimia nervosa (the eating disorders): conditions of interest to the dental practitioner. J Dent. 1996;24(1/2):7–16.

Roberts MW. Oral findings in anorexia nervosa and bulimia nervosa: a study of 47 cases. J Am Dent Assoc. 1987;115(3): 407–410.

Touyz SW, Liew VP, Tseng P, Frisken K, Williams H, Beumont PJ. Oral and dental complications in dieting disorders. Int Eat Disord. 1993;14(3):341–347.

Vestergaard P, Emborg C, Stoving RK, Hagen C, Mosekilde L, Brixen K. Patients with eating disorders. A high-risk group for fractures. Orthop Nurs. 2003;22(5): 325–331.

Woodmansey KF. Recognition of bulimia nervosa in dental patients: implications for dental care providers. Gen Dent. 2000;48(1):48–52.

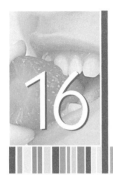

NUTRITIONAL COUNSELING

Introduction

"It's fine for dental hygienists to give out general nutrition information but state laws and licensure regulations draw the line when it comes to giving specific nutrition advice and counsel regarding a specific health condition. For that, oral health care professionals should refer patients to a registered dietitian."

Gail Frank, DrPH, RD[1]

Before getting started with nutritional counseling in the dental office, it is wise to understand the difference between what is expected of dental professionals and what is considered beyond the scope of practice. Dental nutritional counseling was developed to prevent or minimize dental disease and should be the goal in discussing food and diet with patients. Becoming involved in a patient's weight loss or recommending a diet for a specific medical condition is beyond the scope of practice and is better left to physicians or registered dietitians.

What do dental patients know? Most fail to recognize the relationship that nutritional status and eating habits have with their dental health. They don't really understand that what, when, and how they eat can affect their dental health. They do have a vague understanding that sugar causes cavities, but how diet relates to the health of the soft tissues and periodontium is not common knowledge. Teaching the interrelationship between diet and dental health can be as beneficial to the patient and as rewarding to the dental professional as teaching good home care.

There are many well-designed nutritional counseling forms on which to collect diet information; some have different layouts, but all will get you to the same end. If you do not have any forms or are unhappy with the ones you have, most dental and dental hygiene schools are very willing to share what they currently use. If your school or office is open to trying new ideas, visit the school-of-choice's website and navigate to their patient documents or patient forms section. You can also visit the section at the end of this book to see if the nutritional counseling forms and instructions will work for you. Completing them yourself first allows you to get an idea of what you are asking your patients to do and how much time will need to be invested.

Who Can Benefit From Dietary Counseling?

Almost everyone can benefit from learning something new and receiving information that can help improve his or her life. But certain groups are more at risk for nutritional deficiencies that cause or exacerbate dental disease. Knowing which groups to target can ensure that you are helping those with definite need. The following is a list of groups who can benefit from dental nutritional counseling:

- Elderly
  - The elderly are at high risk for dental caries due to dry mouth and increased consumption of simple sugars. Buying food on a fixed income and preparing meals for one person are also complicating factors.
- Teenagers
  - Peer pressure for females to be thin or males to be muscular can create unusual eating habits. Convenience and fast foods are staples in the teen diet, and a balance in food choices is lacking in most cases.
- Bachelors
  - Bachelors are responsible only for themselves; meal planning and preparation is basically nonexistent.
- Adults who diet
  - Specialty diets may raise concerns. The grapefruit diet causes enamel erosion, and the Atkins diet eliminates carbohydrates, causing an imbalance in what is suggested in the Food Pyramid.
- Patients with change in dental health
  - New or recurrent caries as well as exacerbated periodontal disease can be a result of poor snack or meal choices.
- Patients who take medications that cause dry mouth
  - Lack of benefits from saliva can cause an increase in dental caries.

Fitting Dental Nutritional Counseling Into Patient Treatment

In the CDT (Current Dental Terminology) 4 catalog, Nutritional Counseling (code D1310) is listed under Other Preventive Services. Unfortunately, there is no compensation for this procedure provided to dental practices. It falls into the same black hole as fluoride treatments or sealants for a person beyond the age of 14—meaning, provide at the patient's expense. Because time equals money in the dental practice, those in the office may want to provide nutritional counseling during an appointment scheduled for another compensated procedure. Don't confuse an insurance company's lack of compensation for lack of importance. Preventive nutritional counseling is just as important during dental treatment as is reinforcing good home care.

The need for dental nutritional counseling is evaluated during the data collection phase of treatment. Procedures included in the data collection phase are:

1. Medical/Dental History
2. Intra/Extra Oral Exam
3. Gingival Exam
4. PSR/Periodontal Chart
5. Dental Chart
6. Radiographs
7. Nutritional Counseling

Clues to look for in the information collected during data collection include:

- New or recurrent caries
- Tooth loss
- Skin lesions
- Atrophied lingual papillae
- Burning tongue
- Pale or gray mucosa
- Angular chelitis
- Greasy scaly skin around nose
- Inadequately functioning salivary glands
- Difficulty chewing or swallowing
- Ill-fitting dentures
- Sores under appliances
- Loss of lamina dura
- Polypharmacy (multiple medications)
- Erythemic marginal and attached gingiva
- Report of dietary change without physician supervision

If any of the above markers are discovered during data collection, the next step would be to explain the need for nutritional counseling to patients. Give patients a reason for wanting to participate. Explaining the relationship between what you found in their mouth to their diet is a great place to start. Initiating an open dialogue about food and snack selection can give the clinician a peek into the window of patients' eating habits. Once patients realize the connection between their diet and oral concern, their willingness for further investigation usually leads to informed consent. Patients have to be prepared and ready to make a change. Just as telling your patients they need to quit smoking does not always cause the effect you hope for, neither will telling them they need to make a change in their eating habits. They have to buy in to their need for change and be willing to work at it.

Collecting Diet Information

If it is determined that a patient can benefit from nutritional counseling and he or she is willing to participate, the next step is to gather information about his or her eating habits from a diet diary. There are several types of diet diaries to choose from:

- 24-hour recall
- 3-day food record
- 7-day food diary
- Computerized diet assessment

The 24-hour recall works best if desiring a quick inquiry of a patient's eating habits. Simply ask the patient to list all the foods consumed in a 24-hour period, including amount and time of day eaten. Ask if it is typical, and if not, ask what would make it typical. This can be accomplished while providing other treatment, while waiting on the dentist to give an exam, or after the dental charting. If a patient reports sucking on breath mints or hard candy or sipping on four Diet Cokes in a day, you have probably discovered the source of new caries.

The 3- to 7-day diet diary is for a more in-depth study and should include at least 1 day of the weekend. This would require the patient to keep track of the food consumed on a daily basis. Forms should be explained and given to the patient to complete at home and return at the end of the week. After analyzing the content, appoint the patient for a one-on-one counseling session where deficiencies can be explained and suggestions for improvements made.

The computerized diet assessment is more general than dental-related but is good for analyzing the nutrient content of food. There are several software programs that can be purchased or programs online that are helpful if a particular nutrient deficiency is suspected.

Counseling Techniques

When providing one-on-one counseling, there are basically two techniques or interactions:

- The *direct approach* is when you are the dictator and the patient plays a passive role. This is the most **ineffective** method because it is human nature to put up a defense when being told what to do. The directive to quit eating chocolate will fall on deaf ears every time.
- With the *non-direct approach*, the patient is in control and the clinician's role is that of facilitator. This is also referred to the patient-centered technique. It demonstrates respect for what the patient already knows about his or her diet and nutrition, and allows for the patient's input and personal preferences. Change is more apt to happen via this method.

Effective communication is a learned skill. The following are a few tips to make the counseling session more effective:

- Be nonjudgmental of current eating habits, likes, and dislikes.
- Let the patient know you are listening by engaging in good eye contact and nodding your head. Provide feedback as to what you understood them to say.
- Use open body language—no crossed arms, looking down, tapping pencils, swinging legs, or looking around.
- Offer encouragement.
- Sandwich criticism between two positive statements.
- Avoid finger pointing.
- Turn off or turn down the radio and block out external noises.

Intervention in the Dental Office

It is best to counsel your patient in a place that does not invoke anxious feelings. Sitting at a table or counter is better than sitting in the treatment chair.

Seat patients at eye level and provide a surface where you can spread out their counseling forms and write, if necessary. Enhance the learning space with visual aids.

According to the Proctor and Gamble Dental Resource Net Adult Learning Online Program, we retain 75% of what we learn through the sense of vision, 13% through hearing, and 3% through taste and smell. Use the redi-reference card provided with this text as you provide information about healthy eating, snacks, and effect of foods on the oral cavity. Box 16-1 lists examples of visual aids.

When counseling patients, there are two important considerations to keep in mind:

- If you counsel children, the parent has to be present.
- If you counsel a dependent person, the person responsible for his or her diet and preparing and serving his or her food must be present.

BOX 16.1

EXAMPLES OF VISUAL AIDS

- Laminated redi-reference card
- Colorful Pyramid Guides
- Copy of the Guidelines for Americans (or other guidelines)
- Written changes patients have agreed to work on
- Written suggestions on how to make those changes

Analysis of the Diet Diary

After the diet diary is returned and you have had time to examine it, ask yourself the following relative questions:

1. Did the patient meet the serving suggestions for the food groups in the Food Pyramid or other food guide (small or inactive people at the lower end, large or active at the upper end)?
2. Did the patient follow all points of the Dietary Guidelines chosen for them?
3. Did the patient minimize the minutes of acid attack each day?
4. Did the patient include one crunchy food per meal?
5. Did the patient include foods rich in nutrients that keep the periodontium healthy?

When Diet Changes Are Indicated

- Keep it simple.
- Make small changes.
- Offer no more than two suggestions at a time.
- Let the patient choose which two changes they want to work on.

When offering suggestions consider the following:

- Be consistent with current food habits, cultural influences, and regional preferences.
- Consider foods in season.
- Consider cost of food and patient's ability to pay for it.
- Make suggestions for choosing healthy meals at restaurants.
- Suggest changes to reduce cariogenic potential of diet.

Counseling Patients

1. If a specific major nutrient deficiency or excess is discovered, such as protein, carbohydrates, or fats, include the suggestions for increasing the nutrient in the patient's diet listed at the end of those respective chapters.
2. If counseling to reduce cariogenicity of the diet, suggest limiting eating events to three times a day. Reduce snacking unless required for pregnancy or a medical condition.
3. If a patient snacks, recommend fresh fruits, vegetables, popcorn, yogurt, or cheese strips.
4. Cariogenic foods such as retentive starches and sugary foods/liquids should be consumed with meals.

5. When oral hygiene does not follow a meal or snack, suggest that the patient end the eating event with a dairy product, such as cheese or milk, or rinse thoroughly with water.

6. Discourage eating snacks before bed, unless followed by thorough brushing and flossing.

7. Include at least two to four servings of dairy products per day.

8. Drink water between meals and with snacks.

9. The protein and fat in meats can't be metabolized by oral bacteria, so they have no impact on caries risk.

10. Cheese eaten at the end of a meal prevents pH from falling into the critical range.

11. Reinforce eliminating foods perceived as highly retentive.
    - Cookies
    - Crackers
    - Dry cereal
    - Potato chips
    - Caramels, jelly beans, and milk chocolate deliver high levels of sugar to bacteria immediately after the foods are consumed, but only for short periods of time.

12. Educate about the rate of oral clearance.
    - Process of dilution and elimination of food debris from the oral cavity: Normal salivary flow has a caries preventive effect by gradually diluting and removing carbohydrates from the mouth.
    - If meals or snacks are frequent, the calcium and phosphorus in saliva will not have a chance to remineralize the teeth between eating events, and a net demineralization results.

13. Suggest eating foods that stimulate saliva production. Eaten at the end of a meal, they promote the buffering of acids produced by bacteria and clear food from the oral cavity.
    - Celery
    - Sugar-free candy
    - Sugar-free gum
    - Apples

14. Inform about foods that raise the salivary pH.
    - Cheese
    - Chicken
    - Pork
    - Beef
    - Fish
    - Dairy products
    - Chewing gum with xylitol

15. Educate on the physical forms of carbohydrates.
    - Liquid forms: fruit juice, sports drinks, coffee, tea, and soft drinks are in an acidic medium, which further demineralizes teeth.
    - Softening of enamel can occur in as little as 1 hour.
    - Diet sodas lower salivary pH and can demineralize tooth surfaces, independent of bacterial acid production.

16. More suggestions:
    - Replace diet and regular sodas with tea (or fruit juice or water, if patients don't need caffeine).
    - Increase dairy products with yogurt, milk in cereal, or cheese added to a sandwich.
    - Switch to whole grains gradually by combining breads—one piece of white, one piece of whole-wheat—for a sandwich, with the white bread toward the tongue.
    - Gradually switch from whole milk to skim by drinking 2%, then 1%, then $1/2$%, and finally skim milk.
    - Try mixing whole milk with 2% at first.
    - Vegetable and fruit juice is an excellent way to increase fruits and vegetables in the diet.
    - Select large pieces of fruit or take a larger portion of vegetables to increase serving size to equal two for each eating occurrence.
    - Try mixing white and brown rice.
    - Don't eliminate sweets if they're wanted; just eat them with meals.
    - Try a healthy salad with dinner for crunchy food. The fiber will go a long way.
    - Cereal is a quick way to increase grains and dairy products—and it's fortified.
    - Frozen vegetables purchased in bags (don't forget to shake) are great for microwaving.
      - Most people have a tendency to eat the same foods for days, but vegetables in bags allow you to choose something different every day.
      - Just take out what you need and put the bag back in the freezer.

PUTTING THIS INTO PRACTICE

Complete a diet analysis on yourself using the forms provided in the forms section of this book. Follow the instructions for completion, analysis, and counseling. Take notes in a small notepad, noting:
- sections that seemed confusing
- difficulties encountered in maintaining a daily log of foods consumed
- questions that arose as you analyzed the food diary

CHAPTER QUIZ

1. Which of the following methods for collecting data on food intakes would be most practical in a private dental practice?

    a. Nutritional screening questionnaire

    b. 24-hour diet recall

    c. 3- to 7-day food diary

2. The nutritional counseling technique that allows the patient to play an active role in making dietary changes is called:

    a. Direct approach

    b. Nondirect approach

3. Clients over the age of 65 are too old to benefit from making healthy changes in their diets.

    a. True

    b. False

4. At what phase of treatment should the client's nutritional needs be evaluated?

    a. Data collection phase

    b. Initial consultation

    c. Treatment phase

    d. Reevaluation

5. List three effective communication skills.

6. When diet changes are indicated, the clinician should choose two that would benefit the patient most.

    a. True

    b. False

7. The best place to provide dietary counseling is in the treatment chair, where the patient is most familiar with the office.

    a. True

    b. False

Web Resources

Dietitians of Canada www.dieticians.ca

Government Nutrition Site www.nutrition. gov

References

1. Schneidhorst-Olson L. The nutrition balancing act. Access, July 1999.

Suggested Readings

Altschuler B. Nutrition education the role of the dental hygienist. Dental Hyg News 1994;7(3).

Boyd LD, Dwyer JT. Guidelines for nutrition screening, assessment, and intervention in the dental office. J Dent Hyg. 1998;72(4):31–43.

Davis JR, Stegeman CA. The Dental Hygienist's Guide to Nutritional Care. Philadelphia: W. B. Saunders, 1998.

Dreizen S. Dietary and nutritional counseling in the prevention and control of oral disease. Compendium 1989;10(10): 558–564.

Hackett AF, Rugg-Gunn AJ, Appleton DR. Use of dietary diary and interview to estimate the food intake of children. Hum Nutr Appl Nutr. 1983;37(4):293–300.

Hornick B. Diet and nutrition implications for oral health. J Dent Hyg. 2002; 76(1):67–78.

Maclellan DL, Berenbaum S. Client-centered nutrition counseling: do we know what this means? Can J Diet Pract Res. 200364(1):12–15.

Palmer CA. Diet and Nutrition in Oral Health. Upper Saddle River, NJ: Prentice Hall, 2003.

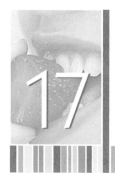

17 SPECIAL NUTRITIONAL NEEDS

Introduction

There are times when you may be required to offer nutritional counseling to patients in special dental circumstances. Some of the dental specialty areas have specific diet concerns, whether it's during treatment or after surgery. Knowing which foods clients should include in their diets will help with their tissue healing and repair.

Diabetes has dental concerns all its own. Clients with this disease can experience both dental caries and periodontal disease, but when counseling them for improvement or prevention of these two dental diseases, it is necessary to keep in mind that diabetics already follow a specialized diet as prescribed by their physician.

Tissue Healing Concepts

Stress, infections, and tissue injuries require an increase in all nutrients to heal the body. When the body is wounded, there is a 25% increase in total calorie requirement for metabolic function to repair and heal. A 12% increase in nutrient requirement is needed for every degree of elevated temperature. When the body needs to repair and heal tissues, there is a daily need for dietary protein. If a deficiency exists, the body will draw from its own structures. Adequate calories are needed to provide the added energy requirement for the repair process.

- 25% increased nutrient needed to repair wounds
- 12% increased nutrient need for every degree of elevated temperature
- Increased need for protein to repair

New Denture Wearer

Imagine having your palate completely covered with a piece of hard plastic. You're trying to bite into a piece of steak with your front teeth and grind with your back teeth, but biting and grinding doesn't work like it used to. Biting feels like the denture can be pulled right out of the mouth along with the food. And grinding is more like smashing and food just doesn't seem to pulverize like before. You have to swallow big chunks of food, which are hard to digest. You wonder why you didn't take better care of your teeth. As the saying goes, you don't appreciate what you have until it's gone.

The new denture patient is dealing with learning to talk and chew in a new way. The dental professional can help them accept the limitations of dentures as they adjust to new "rules" for eating. The following is a list of suggestions that are helpful during this time of change:

- Be aware that food may not taste the same—flavors are masked by the denture.
- Cut regular food into small pieces.
- Chew foods on both sides with the back teeth to prevent tipping of the denture.
- Take small bites and chew slowly.
- Start with soft foods such as eggs, fish, cooked vegetables, and pudding.
- Avoid sticky or very hard foods in the beginning.
- Be careful with food and drinks of hot temperatures, because the denture covers the palate and the heat is not felt until the food is on the way down.

Temperomandibular Joint Disorders

Pain upon chewing can be caused from degeneration of the temperomandibular joint (TMJ). Oftentimes the pain is felt in the ears and temporal region of the skull. Learning to manage the pain while eating is important, and the client collaborates with the dental professional for permanent relief. The following are suggestions that are helpful to alleviate pain while chewing:

- Avoid foods that require you to open wide. Chewing ability may be limited depending on how wide the mouth can be opened.
- If the smallest movements during chewing are painful, try liquid supplements such as Ensure.
- A soft diet is best with eating events divided into several small meals a day so the amount of time needed to chew is limited.

Orthodontic Clients

The main concern about diet and orthodontics is that some foods will displace the brackets, loosen cement under bands, and bend the ligature wire. Plaque accumulates around the appliances and is difficult to remove. If the client has frequent eating episodes of carbohydrates, there is a greater opportunity for acid production and enamel demineralization. The client should be instructed to avoid eating hard or sticky foods and foods with a high carbohydrate content. Most foods can be eaten, but they should be cut into bite-sized pieces. Teeth are usually sore after adjustments so soft foods are tolerated best. Prepare ahead for adjustment days by planning snacks and meals of soft consistency.

Examples of Foods to Avoid:

- Popcorn, nuts, and peanut brittle
- Ice
- Corn on the cob
- Sticky candy such as gummy bears, caramels, taffy
- Any kind of soda
- Corn chips and crisp tacos
- Chewing gum
- Hard bagels, bread, or rolls and pizza crust
- Lemons
- Popcorn kernels
- Hard pretzels
- Biting into whole pieces of fruit with front teeth

Necrotizing Ulcerative Periodontal Diseases

Necrotizing ulcerative periodontal (NUP) disease is a destructive infection that causes necrosis of gingival tissues accompanied by bone loss. Tissues are fiery red, bleed spontaneously, and are extremely painful. Clients will present with elevated temperatures and lymphadenopathy and report a sense of lethargy. Dental treatment consists of aggressive debridement, patient education, and nutritional counseling. The following are diet suggestions that can help the client through the first few critical days:

- Eat liquid or a soft diet for the first few days.
- Avoid all spicy or irritating foods.
- Choose bland foods that feel soothing, such as gelatin and ice cream.
- Eat frequent small meals.
- Drink plenty of fluids.
- Take vitamin/herb supplements as recommended by the DDS.

Periodontal Surgery

Postperiodontal surgery patients will feel significant pain in the area of operation. A wound has been created and will take time to heal. Solid foods can be eaten as long as the client feels comfortable, but if hard to tolerate, soft foods should be eaten for 3 to 4 days until significant healing has occurred. The following is a list of foods to avoid for the first 3 to 5 days after surgery:

- Spicy foods
- Salty foods

- Crunchy or hard foods
- Excessively hot foods and beverages
- Alcoholic beverages

Oral Surgery

Biopsies and other soft tissue wounds should be treated the same as for the periodontal patient. If oral surgery involved tooth extraction, the following are suggestions for eating and drinking:

- Avoid smoking and sucking through a straw because this can dislodge the clot and a dry socket occurs.
- Drink plenty of fluids.
- Eat soft foods during the first 12 to 24 hours.
- Eat your usual diet, but chew on the opposite side of the wound.
- Avoid alcoholic beverages, spicy foods, and hot liquids that may be irritating.

Counseling the Diabetic Client

Millions of people have been diagnosed with diabetes, and there may be millions more who have symptoms but are not yet diagnosed. There are three main types of diabetes:

- Type 1: autoimmune destruction of the cells that produce insulin in the pancreas
- Type 2: impaired insulin function
- Gestational: glucose intolerance during pregnancy (usually a temporary situation)

It is estimated that 20 percent of all adults over the age of 65 are diabetic. Ninety-five percent of diabetics have Type 2 diabetes.[1,2] With figures like these, it is more than likely that dental professionals will treat many diabetics in their practice. The following are some of the risks for an increased incidence of diabetes:

- Prolonged hyperglycemia
- Increase in age
- Obesity
- Long-term lack of physical activity
- Hypertension
- Genetic predisposition
  - African American
  - Hispanic
  - American Indian

For those of us who are healthy, insulin helps our bodies maintain blood sugar levels. Our pancreas secretes insulin when there is an excess of glucose in our blood, such as after a carbohydrate-rich meal, and removes the surplus of glucose, storing it in the muscle and liver as glycogen, where it can be accessed for future energy use. This process of insulin production and glucose removal is ineffective in diabetics.

Dental management of diabetic patients should include:

- Taking a thorough and accurate medical history
- Inquiring about their management of the disease:
  - Oral medications, including dosage and times
  - Eating patterns
  - Insulin injections
  - Frequency of blood glucose readings
- Educating about oral manifestations
  - Oral burning if uncontrolled
  - Increased incidence of periodontal disease
    - Diabetic smokers have a severalfold greater incidence of periodontal disease
  - Xerostomia due to decreased function of parotid gland
    - Increased dental caries at gingival third
    - Angular chelitis and candida infection due to low salivary flow

If providing nutritional counseling in the dental setting for diabetic patients, be reminded that it is beyond the scope of the dental practice to give counseling advice for a specific medical condition. Advising for a diet that can reduce dental caries and periodontal disease are within the bounds of a dental auxiliary and may be necessary if these conditions exist. The following should be included when counseling a diabetic patient:

- Sip on water or chew sugarless gum to help alleviate dry mouth and stimulate saliva flow.
- Follow a balanced diet as prescribed by the physician/dietician to ensure adequate nutrient intake.
- Add a multivitamin to the daily regimen, if not already doing so.
- Include cariostatic foods if allowed in the daily diet.
- Practice thorough daily plaque removal with sulcular brushing and interproximal aids.

PUTTING THIS INTO PRACTICE

Choose two of the special patient groups and make information sheets for your dental practice to give the client as take-home instructions. Include:

- description of the service just provided at the office
- what to expect in the next 24 hours
- suggestions for foods to avoid
- suggestions of foods to include in the diet
- any special oral care instructions

CHAPTER QUIZ

1. Which of the following statements of nutritional advice would you include in your counseling of a patient with a new denture?

    a. Avoid eating anything for the first few days so you can get used to the denture.

    b. Chew food on both sides of the mouth to equalize the chewing forces.

    c. Eat anything you like since caries are no longer a concern.

    d. Avoid all dark-colored foods because they can stain the denture.

2. Which of the following dietary recommendations would you **NOT** want to make to a patient in orthodontic therapy?

    a. Limit sugar consumption to prevent enamel erosion.

    b. Include hard, textured foods for increased salivation.

    c. Chew soft foods after adjustments have been made.

    d. Avoid sticky foods since they can be trapped in the wires.

3. Which of the following special patient groups may require additional liquid nutrient supplements?

    a. Oral surgery

    b. New denture

    c. Orthodontic

    d. Periodontal

    e. TMJ

4. When the body is wounded, there is a _____ increase in total calorie requirement for metabolic function to repair and heal.

    a. 5%

    b. 10%

    c. 25%

    d. 50%

5. When the body needs to repair and heal tissues, there is a daily need for dietary protein.

    a. True

    b. False

6. Which of the following special groups should avoid drinking fluids through a straw for a few days after treatment?

    a. Periodontal surgery

    b. TMJ

    c. NUP

    d. Oral surgery extraction

    e. New denture

7. Which of the following types of diabetes accounts for 95% of all diagnosed cases?

   a. Type 1

   b. Type 2

   c. Gestational

8. Which of the following would be an acceptable nutritional recommendation to a person with Type 2 diabetes?

   a. Eliminate as many carbohydrates from the daily diet as possible

   b. Increase dairy foods and healthy fats to three servings each per day

   c. Increase water intake, sipping throughout the day, and chew on sugarless gum

   d. Increase protein intake to three servings per day

Web References

Fixodent—Information About Dentures http://www.fixodent.com/new_adjust.html

Harvard School of Public Health—Diabetes http://www.hsph.harvard.edu/nutritionsource/diabetes.html

National Diabetes Information Clearing-house (NDIC) www.diabetes.niddk.nih.gov/dm/pubs/eating_ez/index.htm

References

1. Lalla RV, D'Ambrosio JA. Dental management considerations for the patient with diabetes mellitus. JADA 2001;132(10):1425–1432.

2. American Diabetes Association. Position statement on evidence-based nutrition principles and recommendations for the treatment and prevention of diabetes and related complications. Diabetes Care. 2002;25(1):202–212.

Suggested Readings

Ciglar L, Skaljac G, Sutalo J, Keros J, Jankovic B, Knezevic A. Influence of diet on dental caries in diabetics. Coll Anthropol. 2002;26(1):311–317.

Joshipura KJ, Willett WC, Douglass CW. The impact of edentulousness on food and nutrient intake. J Am Dent Assoc. 1996;127(4):459–467.

Lyle D. Diabetes Mellitus. RDH 2003; 54–55.

Marcenes W, Steele JG, Sheiham A, Walls AW. The relationship between dental status, food selection, nutrient intake, nutritional status, and body mass index in older people. J Dent Res. 2001;80(2):408–413.

Riordan DJ. Effects of orthodontic treatment on nutrient intake. Am J Orthod Dentofacial Orthop. 1997;111(5):554–561.

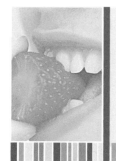

APPENDICES

APPENDIX I

Answers to Chapter Quizzes

Chapter 2
1. b
2. d
3. b
4. a
5. b
6. a
7. b
8. d
9. d
10. b

Chapter 3
1. b
2. c
3. b
4. c
5. b
6. c
7. a
8. d

Chapter 4
1. a
2. d
3. a
4. b
5. b
6. c
7. c
8. d
9. d
10. b

Chapter 5
1. c
2. c
3. d
4. b
5. b
6. c
7. c
8. d
9. a
10. b

Chapter 6
1. a
2. b
3. b
4. b
5. d
6. a
7. b
8. b
9. a
10. d

Chapter 7
1. a
2. b
3. b
4. c
5. d
6. a
7. d
8. b
9. b
10. b

Chapter 8
1. b
2. c
3. b
4. a
5. c
6. b
7. a

Chapter 9
1. c
2. b
3. e
4. a
5. a
6. b
7. a
8. a
9. c
10. d

Chapter 10
1. b
2. a
3. c
4. a
5. b

Chapter 11
1. c
2. b
3. a
4. e
5. b
6. b
7. d
8. c
9. b
10. c

Chapter 12
1. b
2. b
3. b
4. a
5. d
6. c
7. b

Chapter 13
1. c
2. c
3. d
4. a
5. d
6. a
7. a
8. a
9. b
10. e

Chapter 14
1. c
2. a
3. e
4. d

Chapter 15
1. b
2. c
3. b
4. d
5. b
6. b
7. a
8. b

Chapter 16
1. b
2. b
3. b
4. a
5. non-judgmental, open body language, encouraging
6. b
7. b

Chapter 17

1.	b
2.	b
3.	e
4.	c
5.	a
6.	d
7.	b
8.	c

APPENDIX II

Semantics

Essential nutrient = one the body must get by consuming food
Nonessential = a nutrient the body produces
Organic = molecule has a carbon-to-carbon bond or carbon-to hydrogen bond
Inorganic = molecule does not contain carbon
Kilocalorie = different way to say calorie
CHO = carbohydrate
PRO = protein
LIPID = fat
Lysis = split apart
Hydro = water
Peptide = related to protein
Lacto = milk
Ovo = egg

Suffixes

-ase = enzyme
-ose = carbohydrate
-ine = amino acid

Prefixes

mono = one
di = two
tri = three
oligo = two to four
poly = many or more than 10
hyper = over
hypo = under
endo = inside
meso = middle
ecto = outside
Mastication = chewing food
Excretion = elimination of toxic waste via body fluids
Defecation = elimination of solid waste
RDA = recommended daily allowance
RDI = recommended daily intake
Endomorph = small bone structure
Mesomorph = medium bone structure
Ectomorph = large bone structure

Calories/gram

4 calories for each gram of CHO
4 calories for each gram of PRO
9 calories for each gram of FAT
7 calories for each gram of alcohol

APPENDIX III

Forms Index

1. First Food Survey Analysis
2. Second Food Survey Analysis
3. 7-Day Food Survey*
4. 7-Day Snack Survey*
5. 24-Hour Diet Recall
6. Fats Survey
7. High-Nutrient Food List*
8. Low-Nutrient Food List*
9. Nutrition Demographic Survey

*Forms adapted from *Nutrition for Dental Hygienists* by Morris and Knight, 1993.
All forms adapted and created with the help and expertise of Debi Cohn, RDH, Nutritionist.

APPENDIX III.1

First Diet Diary Analysis

Patient's name _____ Student's name _____

1. Does the diet meet the daily requirements of the Food Pyramid? Yes/No

Food Group	Yes	No
Dairy		
Meat		
Fruit		
Vegetable		
Cereals and Grains		
Water		

2. Does the diet meet the recommended Guidelines for Healthy Eating? Address all points.

3. What is the PAP?_____

4. Dental plaque- and decay-producing potential of the diet could be decreased by:

   Eliminating:

   Substituting:

5. Maintenance of healthy periodontium could be improved by including (be specific with foods suggested):

6. What two changes for improvement have been suggested?

   1.

   2.

APPENDIX III.2

Second Diet Diary Analysis

Patient's name _____   Student's name _____

1. Does the second diet diary meet the daily requirements of the Food Pyramid? Yes/No

Food Group	Yes	No	First Diary	Second Diary	Difference
Dairy					
Meat					
Fruit					
Vegetable					
Cereals and Grains					
Water					

2. Does the second diet diary meet the Guidelines for Healthy Eating? Address all points. Has there been an improvement from the last diary?

3. Was there a reduction in the PAP?

First Diet Diary	Second Diet Diary	Difference

4. Were any changes made to maintain healthy periodontium?

5. What two changes for improvement have been suggested?

   1.

   2.

APPENDIX III.3
7-Day Food Survey

Name _____ Date _____

Place a hash mark in the day's box each time you eat a food from a particular food group. Divide by 7 for the week's average.

Group	Serving size	Day 1	Day 2	Day 3	Day 4	Day 5	Day 6	Day 7	Average for week	Recommended	+ or −
Healthy fats and oils	1 T. canola oil, olive oil, peanut oil, cashews, almonds										
Healthy snacks	Fresh fruits, fresh vegetables, cheese, popcorn, nuts										
Meat/substitute	3 oz. meat 3 oz. poultry, fish 1 egg 2 T. peanut butter 1/2 c. cooked legumes										
Dairy	1 c. milk, yogurt 1½ oz. cheese 1/2 c. cottage cheese, frozen yogurt										
Fruits	2–4 medium 3/4 c. juice Source vit. C Source vit. A										
Vegetables	3–5 medium 3/4 c. juice Source vit. C Source vit. A										
Whole grains and fiber	1 slice bread 1/2 English muffin, hamburger bun 3/4 c. dry cereal, grain 1/2 c. rice, pasta 1 muffin, tortilla, roll										
Water	8 oz.										

APPENDIX III.4

7-Day Snack Survey

Name _____   Date _____

Place a hash mark in the box each time you consume a snack between—not as part of—a meal. (Snacks constitute foods eaten at least 20 minutes before or after a meal.) Amount doesn't matter. Add up the minutes and divide by 7 to get the average daily acid production for the week.

Liquid snacks = 30 minutes*
Solid/sticky = 45 minutes*
Slow-dissolving = 60 minutes*
* not scientific—just an estimate of amount of acid attack on enamel
Ideal PAP (potential acid production) = 60 minutes or less each day

Consistency	Day 1	Day 2	Day 3	Day 4	Day 5	Day 6	Day 7
Liquid							
Sweetened coffee/ tea							
Hot chocolate							
Soda							
Flavored milk							
Solid/sticky							
Cookie							
Cake							
Candy—mints, caramel, candy bar							
Pastry, doughnut							
Sugared chewing gum							
Slow-Dissolving							
Lifesavers							
Cough drop							
Sucker							
Breath mint							
Hard candy, candy cane							
Total							

APPENDIX III.5

24-Hour Diet Recall

Name _____   Date _____ M T W Th F S Su

Food	# Servings/Day	Serving Size
Meat/alternative		
Fruit		
Vegetable		
Vitamin C source		
Vitamin A source		
Milk/alternative		
Breads/cereals/grains		
Fats		
Dessert		
Candy/sugar		
Alcohol		
Coffee/tea		
Soda		
Water		
Restaurant meals		
Take-out meals		
Snacks		
Other		

Does this represent a typical day's diet?	Yes	No
Do you take a vitamin/mineral supplement?	Yes	No
Is your present appetite:	Good	Poor
Are you on a special diet?	Yes	No

If so, describe in the box below:

Breakfast

Lunch

Dinner

Snacks (time of day)

APPENDIX III.6

Fats

Place a hash mark next to the listed fat <u>each</u> time you eat it, either in cooking or with a meal.

Monounsaturated

1. Avocado
2. Canola oil
3. Peanut oil
4. Black olives
5. Almonds
6. Cashews
7. Peanuts
8. Pecans
9. Natural peanut butter
10. Olive oil
11. Vinaigrette dressing

Polyunsaturated

1. Low-fat margarine
2. Reduced-fat mayonnaise
3. Walnuts
4. Corn oil
5. Safflower oil

Saturated

1. Bacon
2. Butter
3. Coconut
4. Half & half
5. Whipping cream
6. Sour cream
7. Cream cheese
8. Fat back
9. Shortening or lard

Trans Fats (affects blood vessels same as saturated)

Any food with a label that identifies the following:
1. Hydrogenated
2. Partially hydrogenated

APPENDIX III.7

High-Nutrient Foods

Place a hash mark next to the food each time you eat it, either in a meal or snack during the week.

Meat

1. Water-packed tuna
2. Cod, flounder, salmon
3. Clams, crab, lobster, shrimp
4. Lean pork
5. Scallops
6. Trout
7. Light meat chicken
8. Light meat turkey
9. Veal
10. Lamb roast
11. Flank, round, sirloin steak

Legumes

1. Garbanzo beans
2. Black beans
3. Navy beans
4. Lima beans
5. Kidney beans
6. Green peas
7. Snap-green beans
8. Pinto beans
9. Lentils

Dairy

1. Nonfat yogurt
2. Skim milk
3. Low-fat cottage cheese
4. Low-fat cheese
5. 1% milk

Cereals

1. Grape Nuts
2. Oatmeal
3. Shredded Wheat
4. Cheerios
5. 40% Bran Flakes
6. Special K
7. Crispix

Beverages

1. 8-oz. water
2. Unsweetened tea
3. Fruit juice
4. Vegetable juice

Vegetables

1. Tomato
2. Cucumber
3. Carrots
4. Zucchini
5. Onion
6. Cabbage
7. Corn
8. Potato
9. Green beans
10. Spinach
11. Sweet potato
13. Celery
14. Cauliflower
15. Mushrooms
16. Peppers
17. Summer squash
18. Salad greens
19. Broccoli
20. Corn
21. Other

Grains

1. Pita bread
2. Pumpernickel
3. French bread
4. Raisin bread
5. English muffin
6. Rye bread
7. Wheat bread
8. Other whole-grain bread
9. Whole-grain crackers
10. Whole-grain pasta
11. Brown rice
12. Whole-grain waffle/pancake
13. Whole-grain bagel

Fruits

1. Blackberries
2. Blueberries
3. Pineapple
4. Grapes
5. Apple
6. Peach
7. Plum
8. Pear
9. Strawberries
10. Banana
11. Grapefruit
12. Orange
13. Watermelon
14. Kiwi
15. Cherries
16. Cranberries
17. Melon

APPENDIX III.8

Low-Nutrient Foods

Place a hash mark next to the food <u>each</u> time you eat it, either in a meal or snack during the week.

Meat

1. Ground beef
2. Pork
3. Ham
4. Fish sticks
5. Hot dog
6. Lunchmeat
7. Duck
8. Corned beef
9. Prime rib
10. Spare ribs
11. Pork sausage
12. Fried fish
13. Fried chicken
14. Dark poultry
15. Pork chop
16. Peanut butter

Dairy

1. Whole milk
2. Milkshake
3. American processed cheese
4. Sour cream
5. Half & half
6. Whipping cream
7. Ice cream
8. Cheddar cheese
9. Swiss cheese
10. Cottage cheese
11. Cream cheese

Cereals

1. Fruit Loops
2. Captain Crunch
3. Sugar Pops
4. Lucky Charms
5. Fruity/Cocoa Pebbles
6. Cocoa Puffs
7. Other

Grains

1. White bread
2. Biscuit
3. White rice
4. Semolina pasta
5. Dinner roll
6. Soda crackers
7. Pancakes/waffles
8. Croissant
9. Stuffing
10. Taco shell

Desserts

1. Doughnut
2. Cake
3. Cookie
4. Brownie
5. Pie
6. Snack cakes
7. Ice cream bars
8. Pastry
9. Candy
10. Muffins

Snacks

1. Potato chips/french fries
2. Cheetos
3. Doritos
4. Tostitos
5. Buttered popcorn
6. Slim Jims
7. Smores

Beverages

1. Soda (regular and diet)
2. Sweetened coffee and tea
3. Lemonade
4. Punch
5. Kool-Aid
6. Hot chocolate
7. Chocolate milk
8. International coffee mixes
9. Alcohol

Condiments

1. Salt
2. Sugar
3. Syrup
4. Honey
5. Jelly/jam
6. Butter/margarine

Vegetables

1. Any in cream sauce
2. Au gratin
3. Fried

APPENDIX III.9
Nutrition Survey

Name _____   Date _____

1. Do you eat approximately the same time every day?	Yes	No
2. Do you eat most of your meals in a hurry/on the go?	Yes	No
3. Do you eat alone?	Yes	No
4. Does your religion or culture influence your diet?	Yes	No
5. Have you recently gained or lost at least 10 pounds?	Yes	No
If so, please explain_____		
6. Have you been on a diet in the last 3 months?	Yes	No
If so, list type of diet_____		
7. Do you experience any pain when eating?	Yes	No
8. Do you have any chewing or swallowing difficulty?	Yes	No
9. Do you suffer from chronic indigestion?	Yes	No
10. Have you been told you have gastrointestinal disease?	Yes	No
11. Do you avoid certain foods?	Yes	No
If so, explain_____		
12. Do you take any kind of medication—prescribed or OTC?	Yes	No
If so, please list_____		
13. Do you suffer from a chronic dry mouth?	Yes	No
14. Do you have frequent sores in your mouth?	Yes	No
15. Are your gums red and puffy, and do they bleed easily?	Yes	No
16. Do you eat between-meal snacks?	Yes	No
17. Do your snacks consist of sugar?	Yes	No
18. Do you eat foods with a sticky consistency?	Yes	No
19. Do you drink soft drinks?	Yes	No
If so, how many per day? _____regular _____diet		
20. Do you use tobacco?	Yes	No
21. Do you drink alcohol?	Yes	No
If so, how many ounces per day?_____		
22. Do you drink tea or coffee every day?	Yes	No
With cream/cremora?	Yes	No
With sugar/sweetener?	Yes	No
23. Do you take a multivitamin?	Yes	No
24. Do you take any herbal supplements?	Yes	No
If so, please list_____		
25. Do you drink at least 8 glasses of water a day?	Yes	No
26. Do you know your HDL, LDL, and triglyceride levels?	Yes	No
If so, please list _____		

27. Is your blood pressure within normal range?   Yes   No

    If not, please explain_____

28. Do you get aerobic exercise three to five times per week?   Yes   No

29. Do you eat red meat more than three times per week?   Yes   No

30. Are you familiar with trans fats?   Yes   No

31. Do you know the difference between saturated,

    monounsaturated, and polyunsaturated fats?   Yes   No

32. Do you frequently eat meals out at a restaurant?   Yes   No

33. How often do you eat fast foods? _____

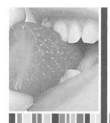

INDEX

Page numbers in *italics* denote figures; those followed by a "t" denote tables; those followed by a "b" denote boxes